Comments on *Kidney Transplants Exp*

'I wish I had had access to a similarly i............. ....
encountered kidney failure 20 years ago.'

Deborah Duval, Editor, Kidney Life

'As the husband of a transplant patient I found the chapter on transplant
failure emotive, but factual and true in its assessment of the community's
ability to support such an event. I would not change it.'

Bob Dunn, National Kidney Federation

'It is very readable and I really enjoyed the style of writing and the
patient scenarios to illustrate particular issues.'

Lisa Burnapp, Consultant Nurse: Living Donor Renal Transplantation,
Guy's and St Thomas's NHS Foundation Trust

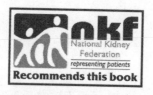

Recommends this book

The National Kidney Federation (NKF) is a charity representing all kidney patients in the United Kingdom, it is run by Kidney patients for Kidney patients. The Federation campaigns for increased renal provision and improved treatment. The charity also provides national services to assist all kidney patients.

Publications recommended by the NKF have to be of a high standard and easily readable, the recommendation is not given lightly and is highly prized. The NKF recommendation of this book was made at the time of its publication and has to be renewed at subsequent prints in order to retain the NKF endorsement and recommendation. Further information about the NKF and books it recommends can be found on its website www.kidney.org.uk.

Kidney Transplants Explained

Dr Andy Stein, MD, FRCP
*Consultant Nephrologist and General Physician,
University Hospitals Coventry and Warwickshire NHS Trust*

Dr Rob Higgins, MD, FRCP
*Consultant Nephrologist, University Hospitals
Coventry and Warwickshire NHS Trust*

Janet Wild, RGN
*Clinical Education Manager, Baxter Healthcare Ltd,
Newbury, Berkshire*

CLASS PUBLISHING · LONDON

Printing history
First published 2008

10 9 8 7 6 5 4 3 2 1

The authors and publishers welcome feedback from the users of this book. Please contact the publishers.

Class Publishing, Barb House, Barb Mews, London W6 7PA, UK
Telephone: 020 7371 2119
Fax: 020 7371 2878 [International +4420]
email: post@class.co.uk
www.class.co.uk

The information presented in this book is accurate and current to the best of the authors' knowledge. The authors and publisher, however, make no guarantee as to, and assume no responsibility for, the correctness, sufficiency or completeness of such information or recommendation. The reader is advised to consult a doctor regarding all aspects of individual health care.

A CIP catalogue record for this book is available from the British Library

ISBN 9781859591932

Illustrated by Darren Bennett and David Woodroffe

Edited by Richenda Milton-Thompson

Designed and typeset by Martin Bristow

Printed and bound in Finland by WS Bookwell, Juva

This book is dedicated to those pioneering patients who take part in transplantation research. Without them, no progress could be made.

Contents

Foreword

The National Kidney Federation (NKF) regards transplantation as the 'gold standard' treatment for patients with established renal failure (ERF). It has taken a long battle by the NKF to get the government to recognise that, for most patients, transplantation is a better option compared with dialysis, and that there are also benefits for the NHS and the Treasury.

Now things are changing. The emphasis is at last on transplantation, even pre-dialysis transplantation in some cases. The Federation is gratified to see this turnaround – although it remains determined to press for a very large increase in the numbers of operations performed.

For a renal patient, transplantation is an enormous decision, and one that needs to be taken carefully and with an informed perspective.

The NKF realised that no book currently existed specifically to explain the myriad of issues in a clear and concise way. So it asked Class Publishing to commission such a book and made NKF staff members available to assist. By approaching Andy Stein, Rob Higgins and Janet Wild to be the authors, Class Publishing pulled off a master stroke. This excellent book is the result.

Timothy F Statham, OBE
Chief Executive, National Kidney Federation

Authors' Acknowledgements

Andy Stein and Janet Wild have written three successful books about kidney failure, two of which are primarily for patients with the disease. For this book Rob Higgins, who has also authored a number of patient information books, joined the team. We hope our combined efforts have produced something worthwhile and readable.

Kidney Transplants Explained would never have been written, however, without the insistence of two people: Tim Statham from the National Kidney Federation, who had the original idea for the book, and Dick Warner from Class Publishing, who pursued and cajoled the three of us to put it together.

There are many others 'behind the scenes' whose support, encouragement and advice have been more valuable than they could ever imagine.

For Andy, the mentorship and inspiration he received from the late Professor John Walls, has in no small way enabled him to 'just do it' (the Prof's motto). Andy's colleagues at the University Hospitals of Coventry and Warwickshire must be thanked for allowing him time to write. Finally, Andy would like to thank his family for everything: his partner Emma and their two children, Poppy and Isaac; and his mother Dr Gillian Matthews.

Rob gives special thanks to his partner Pam, to Titus, and to Janet Windsor who read some of the chapters in early draft form.

For this particular book, Janet took advice from the brilliant nephrologists Simon Davies and Alastair Hutchison. Although they may have been be unaware of this, they helped enormously by asking questions and discussing the controversies about the treatment of kidney patients in the UK. Invaluable support came from her husband Chris, who became for many months, once more, a 'book widow', and their two children Archie and Charlie.

Darren Bennett and David Woodroffe are thanked for their clear diagrams, and Mr FT Lam for advising exactly where to put the incisions for a nephrectomy. We also thank Judith Wise for her tireless work in marketing the book.

Huge thanks go to Richenda Milton-Thompson, our magnificent editor, who has diplomatically and tirelessly co-ordinated the contributions of three wilful authors. Throughout, she has insisted on factual accuracy and clear writing for our readers.

Introduction

A successful kidney transplant is generally a more effective treatment for kidney failure than dialysis. This is because a well-functioning transplanted kidney can do all the jobs your own kidneys could do before they failed, whereas dialysis really does only a couple of these jobs. This means that people who have a well-functioning kidney transplant often feel fitter than they did on dialysis. Given the costs of providing dialysis, transplants are now also recognised as being a cost-effective treatment, as well as one that contributes greatly to quality of life.

Not all kidney patients are suitable for transplantation, however, and not all suitable patients are suitable all the time.

It is important to be properly prepared for a transplant. The aim of this book is to help you with that preparation by answering many of the questions you might want to ask about transplants. We hope you will find it useful if you are thinking about having a transplant yourself, if you are living with a transplanted kidney, if someone close to you has (or is thinking about having) a kidney transplant, or if you are thinking about donating one of your kidneys to someone else.

If you have established renal failure (ERF), a successful kidney transplant can really restore your quality of life. There is no doubt that, for the right patient at the right time, a transplant is the best treatment option. A 'good' transplant provides about 60% of the function of two normal kidneys (compared with only about 5% from either type of dialysis). At this level of kidney function, your blood creatinine level will be under $150\,\mu mol/L$ – this means that even with a 'stable' transplant, you will still have chronic kidney disease at Stage 3 (CKD3A). Appendix 1 gives you more information about what different creatinine levels actually mean. In other words, even a transplant that is working well does not cure established renal failure, or get rid of the underlying disease that has caused it. But it should improve your health and your general quality of life considerably.

The most obvious advantage of a transplant if you have kidney failure is that it gives you freedom from dialysis. If your transplant works well, dialysis will become a thing of the past. You will also find you can say goodbye to those tough restrictions on how much you can drink (we are talking fluid, rather than alcohol though!) and just what types of food you can eat. You may also be able to stop taking some of your medications, including erythropoiesis-stimulating agents (ESA), and phosphate binding tablets such as Calcichew. However, you will need drugs to stop your body rejecting the kidney (see Chapter 8) and may need treatment to keep your blood pressure and cholesterol levels low.

Not all renal units in the UK have a 'transplant centre' with a surgeon who performs the transplant operations. However all renal units do have a transplant programme and offer the same opportunities to all patients. Even if they don't offer transplant surgery, they will have a transplant team, usually made up of a doctor and a nurse/transplant coordinator. Most renal units also have a link to the nearest transplant centre. You do not have to have your transplant there. If you prefer another centre, you can be ask to be referred to that centre.

Transplant surgeons are responsible for the transplant operation. They put the new kidney into the patient and connect it to the veins, arteries and ureter. Once this 'plumbing job' has been done, who leads the care of the patient, after that, varies from unit to unit. Either way, at some point, you are handed back to the kidney doctor or 'nephrologist' (like Rob or Andy), in your home renal unit. The kidney doctor is the person who will decide which anti-rejection drugs need to be taken, what their dose should be and will treat any episodes of rejection. Some surgeons in the transplant centre keep control of the patients' care until discharge, others for up to 6 months. This partly depends on the policy of your own renal unit – for example, a surgeon might send back a similar patient early to one unit, and later to another.

Most people who have had a transplant feel better and have more energy than they did on dialysis. They are better able to cope with a job, and many find their sex lives improve. Women are more likely to get pregnant and have a healthy baby.

It is important to recognise that there can be downsides too. Some people who have been on haemodialysis long term have built up valuable social networks around their dialysis sessions, and they may find the change to their routine leaves them lost and lonely. They may also find they lose benefits such as Disabled Living Allowance (DLA). Having a gap of several years in the CV is helpful to no one. So if you are in this situation, you may find that going back to work after a transplant does not make such a positive difference to your financial position as you might hope.

There are patients who, after careful consideration, choose to stay on dialysis. This decision must be respected. It is also important, however, that people who have taken this option are aware that they can change their mind at a later date.

Our aim is to help you understand the process of workup for a transplant, the operation itself, and how to look after the kidney. There is a major focus on living transplantation, as more and more kidneys are now coming from living donors in the UK. We also discuss the postcode lottery, as it applies to transplantation. Like our previous books, *Kidney Transplants Explained* is hard-hitting, describing the disadvantages (and complications) of transplantation, not just the advantages.

We hope you like the book.

Andy Stein, Rob Higgins *and* **Janet Wild**
Coventry and Saddleworth, 2008

1
Suitable for transplant?

In this chapter, we discuss the things that are important to consider before having a kidney transplant. We look at who is likely to be offered a transplant and what you can do if you are not on the transplant waiting list.

Currently in the UK, the majority (about two thirds) of kidneys for transplantation are donated from people who have died (called a *deceased donor transplant* or a *cadaveric transplant*). The remaining third come from living donors. Most healthy people have two kidneys and, providing they are both functioning well, it is possible to remain healthy with just one of them. For this reason, people can donate one of their kidneys while they are still alive. The 'waiting list' for kidney transplants (see Chapter 3) is for people who are waiting for a deceased donor transplant.

WHO CAN HAVE A TRANSPLANT?

About half of all people with established kidney failure are likely to benefit from a transplant, provided a suitable donor kidney can be found. Patients who will probably not be considered suitable include anyone with serious heart or lung disease, or with some types of cancer.

Most kidney units do not have an upper age limit for kidney transplantation. Patients are considered on suitability (i.e. how much difference having a transplant is likely to make to their health) rather than age. However, having said that, most units would think very seriously before transplanting a patient over 70 years old, or indeed before taking a kidney from a living donor over this age.

The main reason for limiting transplants among older patients is that they often do not tolerate the operation very well. Also, the drugs that are needed after a transplant (see Chapter 8) can be too strong for people who are older or in fragile health. However, the chance of getting onto the transplant list varies from hospital to hospital. This may be due to differences in the criteria used to decide whether someone is fit for a transplant, and differences in doctors' points of view. Some doctors are more inclined to give as many people as possible the chance of a transplant. Others feel that since donor kidneys are in short supply, younger and fitter people (i.e. the ones they believe are likely to benefit the most) should be given preference.

NOT ENOUGH KIDNEYS: WHO SHOULD HAVE PRIORITY?

Entry to the transplant list continues to be a subject for debate and discussion. Should anyone who wants a transplant be able to go on the transplant list, or should the list be restricted to younger and fitter people? Some doctors think that transplants should be given to younger and fitter people only. This is because there are never enough kidneys for transplantation. Many doctors feel that older people, and those with serious problems such as heart disease, should remain on dialysis. They argue that this not only makes financial sense for the Health Service (older and/or weaker patients might not tolerate the transplant operation well, resulting in a long hospital stay), but it is also fairer to the donor and the donor family. They would argue that offering the transplant kidney to a younger, fitter person means it is likely to stay working and working well for longer.

On the other hand, some doctors will give the chance of a transplant to older people and to some people with other medical problems such as serious heart or lung disease. Research shows that many people will live longer with a transplant – and everyone is likely to have a better quality of life – than would be the case if they had stayed on dialysis. So, it is perhaps only fair that as many people as possible have the chance of a longer and better quality life.

The trouble is that while the number of people waiting for a transplant is rising year after year, the number of deceased donor kidneys for transplantation that are available each year increases very little if at all. That is why younger, fitter people are often given priority when a kidney becomes available for transplant.

Your doctor will assess your fitness for a transplant and everything will be taken into consideration, including any long-term problems that you have with your heart, circulation or breathing. If the doctors think that you have a higher than average risk of dying within a year of having the operation, you are unlikely to be eligible for a transplant. You do have a right to challenge this decision though. Anyone who feels that they have been unfairly excluded from going onto the transplant list, or who has been removed from the list unfairly, or without being given a proper explanation, should discuss the issue with their own doctor. You also have a right to request a second opinion. So, if you are unhappy with your doctor's view, do ask for one.

Don't feel embarrassed at the thought of 'offending' your doctor and don't be intimidated by your doctor's reaction. This is your life and your health. You need to be confident and feel involved with any decisions that are made. If you do find the idea of approaching your doctor difficult, why not have a word with one of the renal nurses instead? Alternatively, you can discuss your concerns with your GP who will be able to refer you to a different unit.

FITNESS FOR TRANSPLANTATION

Before you can actually have your kidney transplant, you will need to have some tests to make sure that you are fit enough to cope with the operation. These tests may include:

- An electrocardiogram (ECG, an electric recording of your heartbeat);

- A chest X-ray;

- An echocardiogram (ECHO, an ultrasound or sound-wave picture of your heart);

- An 'exercise test' (a test in which you have to walk on a moving walkway, to test your fitness, and stress your heart).

Some kidney units also insist that kidney patients who have diabetes are given more detailed heart tests. These might include a cardiac catheter test (a special X-ray picture of the heart). This cardiac test has some risk, causing death in 1 in 1,000 patients and increasing the risk of complete kidney failure in some patients who are not yet on dialysis. The exercise tests and cardiac catheter may be replaced, over the next few years, by CT scans of the heart, since newer CT scanners are able to take very detailed images.

Transplantation at most centres is generally restricted to people who are physically quite fit, and who have a good chance (about 90%, or 9 out of 10) of being alive a year after the transplant. Many doctors feel this is an appropriate level of risk, given the availability of transplant organs. However, this approach excludes many people from the transplant list, and a high proportion of these would be delighted to have the opportunity to receive a transplant.

One example of how some transplant centres are trying to make kidney transplantation available to more people is by insisting that people who are overweight lose weight before they can go onto the transplant list. This is also the case for people wanting to have a living donor transplant and, in these cases, both the donor and the recipient should be a healthy weight before surgery.

The British Transplantation Society (BTS) has guidelines designed to help people who are less fit to have a transplant. These guidelines have been developed in conjunction with patients and their families. The Renal Association (the UK's society of kidney doctors) is also developing guidelines that should be available in 2008/9.

The BTS recommends that some patients who have serious medical conditions that could lower their chances of survival could receive a transplant from a living donor rather than going onto the transplant list. This would also help to make the system fair by using the scarce kidneys donated from deceased donors for transplants in people who have a higher chance of survival.

MIKE: GETTING ONTO THE WAITING LIST

Mike is a 62-year-old ex-postman who has been on peritoneal dialysis at home for the past two years. He has been coping well and has had no problems with the treatment although he took early retirement shortly after he started dialysis.

When Mike was 56 he was diagnosed with cancer of the bladder. He was given chemotherapy, which worked well and required no further treatment. He has now been free from the disease for five years.

At the time Mike started dialysis he was told that he would not be eligible for a transplant because he had recently suffered from cancer. This was very disappointing to start with, but now that he is settled on dialysis and his cancer has not come back, he feels that it is time for the decision to be reconsidered.

Mike speaks to his specialist kidney doctor at his next routine dialysis clinic appointment. His doctor thinks that it might be possible for Mike to go onto the transplant waiting list. Alternatively, he might be able to have a kidney donated by a friend or relative. The doctor organises the tests that will help to decide whether Mike is fit enough for the operation and asks him to speak to his close family about the possibility of someone donating a kidney.

Following these tests, Mike is told that he is fit and able to go onto the waiting list for a deceased donor kidney. One of his daughters is also having tests to see whether she might be able to donate a kidney to him.

The recommendation from the BTS is that people should be expected to be alive for at least two years after the transplant. Although life expectancy for these people would be the same if they stayed on dialysis or if they had a transplant, most would experience a much better quality of life with a well-functioning transplant. So even though they might not live any longer, they would feel better and be able to live more normally.

TESTING FOR INFECTIONS

In addition to these 'fitness' tests, patients also need to be tested for a number of viral infections before going on the transplant list. These include:

- HIV (the virus that causes AIDS);
- Hepatitis B;
- Hepatitis C;
- Cytomegalovirus (CMV);
- Epstein-Barr virus (EBV).

People should also have their level of immunity to the chicken pox virus, herpes zoster, tested. This determines the treatment they may get if they come into contact with a chicken pox case in the future.

It is important to test for these viruses because they may be dormant ('sleeping', causing no symptoms) in a patient's body. After the transplant, they may be 'woken up' and cause illness. This is especially true of CMV and EBV.

If someone does test positive for HIV, or for the viruses that cause hepatitis B or hepatitis C, it may not be possible for them to have a transplant. However, some people with these viruses are able to receive a transplant after further tests, and possibly treatment with drugs to reduce the level of virus in the body. Even then, they may still be able to get a transplant. But it does mean that the doctors will have to plan the operation extremely carefully and make sure they keep a close eye on the situation afterwards.

Patients who refuse to have any of these tests, including the test for HIV, will definitely not be able to have a transplant.

Everyone should have the opportunity to discuss kidney transplantation in more detail with an expert. A transplant surgeon and a specialist nurse will be able to talk about many of the issues that may concern you if you are about to go onto the transplant list. Talking about the issues beforehand can be valuable as it often helps to make feelings and opinions about the transplant much clearer before it happens. Transplants from deceased donors often happen in a rush, leaving little time to consider all of the issues involved. So, the more you have been able to explore and find out beforehand, the better.

WHAT IF YOU HAVE A SERIOUS VIRUS?

Some transplant units are less keen than others on transplanting patients who test positive for hepatitis B, hepatitis C or HIV. This is because many doctors think the immunosuppressant drugs that people need to take after a transplant, to stop the body rejecting the kidney, will make the virus worse. Certainly, this can happen. This is more likely to concern the doctors than any worry that they might get infected themselves while performing the operation.

With modern drugs, however, patients with these viruses can live as long as someone with diabetes for example. Few people would say that patients with diabetes should not receive a transplant. So, doctors in some transplant centres believe that people with hepatitis or HIV should be given their chance to receive a kidney transplant, especially if they have a friend or relative willing to donate a kidney.

If you have one (or more) of these viruses, and you are turned down by your local transplant centre, why not ask for a second opinion from another unit?

GETTING INFORMATION EARLY

The surgeon or transplant coordinator can explain in detail what happens during the operation and afterwards. They can also help you talk through any concerns you might have about the success of the transplant, the risks and the benefits, and how it will affect your life in ways that are unique to you. Indeed, some 'medically suitable' patients prefer to stay on dialysis, rather than undergo a transplant, because they feel well and are able to live their life to the full in spite of being on dialysis. If this is what you decide, it is important you understand the decision is reversible. You can change your mind and go onto the transplant list at a later date.

Not all centres are good at giving patients all the information they need, but there are other ways of finding out what is likely to happen if you have a transplant. Perhaps the most valuable way is through talking to other patients. This can be very helpful, especially for living donor pairs. The National Kidney Federation (NKF) also offers help and information for both donors and recipients. See their website address in Appendix 2.

GETTING ONTO THE LIST

If results of all your tests are satisfactory, you can then go onto the national waiting list for a deceased donor transplant (see Chapter 3), or be considered for a transplant from a living donor. In most transplant centres throughout the UK, patients have to see the transplant surgeon before being placed on the list. This enables the surgeon to meet and examine the patient, and to explain more about the operation and what you should expect afterwards.

You will find you can't just go onto the list automatically. It can take longer than you might expect to get all the tests and checks done. However, some transplant centres are now using the national 18 week waiting time as a target for how long it should take to prepare patients to go onto the transplant waiting list. The same 18 week target is also being used for preparing patients and their donors for a living transplant.

KEY FACTS

❶ About half of all kidney patients are suitable for a transplant, but not all kidney patients are suitable all the time.

❷ Patients who want to have a transplant need to be assessed for their suitability. This is called a 'transplant work-up'.

❸ The transplant work-up shouldn't take any longer than 4 months.

❹ The main reasons for people being unsuitable for a transplant include serious heart or lung disease, serious forms of cancer, or obesity.

❺ There are guidelines that are designed to help less suitable patients to get a transplant.

2
Matching a kidney to a patient

This chapter describes the process of 'matching up' kidneys with people who need them. It looks at blood groups and tissue typing, and considers other factors that may affect how well a transplant kidney will work for you.

For a kidney transplant to be successful, it is necessary to prevent your body's immune system (natural defence system) attacking the kidney and rejecting it (see Chapter 5 for a description of the rejection process). Rejection is caused by differences between your tissues and those of the donor. The closer the match, the less likely rejection is to occur; and tissue matching is used to help allocate kidneys from deceased donors to the most suitable patient. But, even with good matching, rejection is possible

This is why you will be given drugs that suppress the immune system after the operation. As modern drugs are effective at treating rejection, transplants can often be performed successfully even if there is not a very close match between tissue types. This allows living donor transplants between people who care about each other, but are not related by blood (a husband and wife, for example) to go ahead routinely.

To work out the match between you and a kidney donor, doctors need to carry out a number of tests so that they can work out your blood group (see opposite) and tissue type (see page 14). The results will then be checked against the results of similar tests carried out either on an available kidney from a deceased donor, or on a living person who is considering giving you one of their kidneys.

MATCHING THE BLOOD GROUP

The blood group is an inherited characteristic of red blood cells. Cells are the building blocks of nature, and there are two main types in the blood: red cells, that carry oxygen, and white cells, that primarily fight infection. Your blood group stays the same throughout your life. There are four main blood groups: A, B, AB and O. Group O is the most common, followed by group A – except in Asian people, in whom group B is the most common.

Your blood group depends on whether or not you have certain substances called antigens (types of protein) in your body. Two different antigens – called A and B – determine a person's blood group. If you have these antigens, they will be inside your kidney, not just on your blood cells. If you only have antigen A, your blood group is A. If you only have antigen B, your blood group is B. If you have both antigen A and antigen B, your blood group is AB. If you have neither of these antigens, your blood group is O.

Your immune system will attack any cells that have a foreign antigen on their surface. This means that you can only receive a transplant kidney if your blood group is compatible with the donor's blood group, as follows:

Patient	Donor
Group O	Group O
Group A	Group A or group O
Group B	Group B or group O
Group AB	Any group (O, A, B, or AB)

The cross-match

This is a blood test you will be given after you have been called into hospital to receive a transplant from a deceased donor, or while you are preparing to receive a transplant from a living donor. It tests whether the kidney you are being offered is likely actually to work for you.

A cross-match is done by mixing a sample of your blood with blood cells from the donor. If there is no reaction (i.e. if your blood does not start attacking the donor's cells), it is assumed that you will be less likely to reject the new kidney when it is transplanted. This is called a negative cross-match, and means that the operation can go ahead. So a negative cross-match is a good thing.

If you are having a deceased donor transplant, the cross-match is done quickly, just before the operation. If you are having a living donor transplant, it is done sometime during the work-up process; then repeated 2–3 days before the operation, just to make sure nothing has changed. If the cross-match is positive at this stage, your operation will need to be delayed while the doctors find out why.

If the cross-match is positive (i.e. if there is a reaction between your blood and the donor's cells), the transplant is unlikely to go ahead and you will go back on the waiting list or you may find an alternative living donor.

This can be very disappointing, but it is much better to carry on with dialysis for a while than to be given a kidney that doesn't work, and which may make you extremely ill. There are special circumstances where a transplant can go ahead after a positive cross-match (see page 59). If your blood contains antibodies against other people's tissue types, it is more likely that the cross-match will be positive. Some people have a great many such antibodies, which may leave them with very little chance of ever receiving a deceased donor kidney with a negative cross-match. Indeed, the national kidney allocation scheme computer has records of the anti-bodies patients do have, so they will not be offered kidneys that are bound to give rise to a positive cross-match.

MATCHING THE TISSUE TYPE

A sample of your blood will be needed, along with a sample from the donor kidney or potential living donor. These samples will be tested to determine the tissue types. This tissue typing test reveals your genetic make-up (a type of 'genetic fingerprint'). It will also reveal the genetic make-up of the donor.

The tissue type is an inherited set of characteristics (antigens) on the surface of most cells. It stays the same throughout your life. You have only one tissue type (just as you only have one blood group), but your tissue type is made up of many different tissue type characteristics. Six of these are used for matching purposes. It is also referred to as 'HLA type'.

There are three main sorts of tissue type characteristic, called A, B and DR. Everyone has two of each (one from each parent) – making six in all. There are many different types of A, B and DR characteristic. In fact there are around 40 different versions of each A, B and DR characteristic. This means that there are hundreds of different possible tissue types. So, for example, a tissue type could be A1/A2, B7/B8, DR2/DR3.

As there are so many possible tissue types, matching tissue types is rather more complicated than matching blood groups. However, basically the more of the characteristics that are the same for the patient and the donor kidney, the better the chances will be that the transplant kidney will work.

Given the large number of tissue type possibilities, it is very unusual to get an exact match. This is sometimes described as a '6 out of 6 match', or a 'full-house match' between a patient and donor. But, confusingly, most doctors actually use a negative terminology, i.e. calling it a 'zero mismatch'. In general, most transplant centres will offer a deceased donor transplant if the patient and donor have three or more of the six tissue

---

IS TISSUE TYPE MATCHING REALLY THAT IMPORTANT?

Due to the relatively small advantage of tissue type matching in modern transplant success rates, some doctors think it is not worth the effort.

Theoretically, the better the match, the more likely it is that the body will accept the kidney 'as its own' and not try to reject it. This would lead you to think that the more characteristics that match, the better. So a '4 out of 6 match' would be better than a '2 out of 6 match'. In fact, there is little benefit to having 1–4 of these antigens matching (the same). Only when 5 or 6 antigens are the same, is there much benefit to matching. It is necessary to be a bit more careful for deceased donor transplantation, but we still don't need as close a match as was thought previously to be the case (due to improvements in drug treatments for patients after transplant).

It may be that other factors are more important than tissue type matching to the success of a transplant. For example, we know that the cold ischaemia time (the time that a transplant kidney is out of the body) affects the long-term survival of the kidney. Not surprisingly, the shorter the time a kidney is outside the donor, the fresher it is and, on average, the better it will work. But cold ischaemia time doesn't really make a difference to the success of the transplant if the donor and the recipient are well matched. It's really only a problem when there is a mismatch. In such cases, it may be better to give a deceased donor kidney taken from a donor in Bath, to a recipient, say, in Bristol; rather than send it up to Dundee, to a slightly better matched patient.

What this tends to mean in practice is that transplant centres that are prepared to give a transplant to less well matched patients may get less good results. But you may be more likely to get on the waiting list, and indeed to get a kidney for transplantation, in just those units.

---

type characteristics in common, and there is at least one common DR characteristic. In terms of the expected function of the transplant, it is more important that the DR characteristics are matched than the A or B types. So, for example, a transplant might be offered in the following situation:

Patient:	A1/A2	B7/B8	DR2/DR7
Donor:	A1/A3	B7/B12	DR2/DR7

As the A1, B7, DR2 and DR7 characteristics are the same in this example, it would be called a '4 out of 6 match, with both DR antigens matching'.

Just to confuse matters, again using the negative terminology, doctors actually talk about the number of antigens that don't match – i.e., this would be called a '2 antigen mismatch' because A3 and B12 are not present in the patient.

Under the new matching scheme introduced in 2006, the hospital doesn't get the option to offer kidneys, or only rarely, so the matching decision is made by the national computer.

In fact, there is no guarantee that even a '6 out of 6' antigen match will not be rejected. This is because the blood group and tissue type are not the only cell surface characteristics that are important. Unfortunately, as yet, the other important characteristics have not all been identified.

THE PERFORMANCE OF UK TRANSPLANT CENTRES

Not all UK renal units have a transplant centre. Those that do may have a special interest in one or more aspects of transplantation such as living donor transplants, immunology research, antibody incompatible transplants or pancreas transplants. Those renal units that don't operate a transplant service have the opportunity to refer their patients to any of the transplant centres in the UK. This gives them an opportunity to chose to send their patients to a centre close by their own hospital, or one further afield that has good results in one area or another. The number of referrals from other renal units that a transplant centre receives might have some impact upon their results. You have a right to ask the doctors, nurses or managers about the performance of the centre that will do your transplant. You may want to know:

- How many transplant operations the centre does each year.
  The more operations that are performed, the more experience the hospital will have.

- How long, on average, do transplanted kidneys last in patients from the unit? This precise information is not available on the UKT website; what is available are the percentages of transplant failures and deaths at 1 and 5 years after the transplant. For a summary, see Table 2.1.

- However, you also need to be aware that there are a number of different factors that affect simple percentages. As you can see from Table 2.1, people who have a transplant in Bristol seem to have a better chance that their kidney will still be working 5 years after the operation than those who had a transplant in Plymouth but there could be a number of reasons for this difference. The transplant centre in Bristol may have strict criteria for the types of people going onto the transplant waiting list, whereas the centre in Plymouth may be prepared to transplant patients who are less fit or who have other problems that might affect the success of their transplant.

- How many of the transplants are carried out using kidneys from living donors.

- If you are a living donor, will you be reimbursed for donor loss of income and any expenses incurred? Generally, your Primary Care Trust should pay your expenses, but your transplant coordinator should be able to put you in touch with the relevant contact for claiming these. If your PCT says they have no duty to reimburse you, you should contact the NKF (address in Appendix 2) for advice on how best to proceed.

You have a right to know the answers to these questions, and the information is freely available on the UK Transplant website (see Appendix 2). This website is updated every year.

The number of transplants from either deceased or living donor transplants does vary considerably from one centre to another around the country. The survival rates also vary, but by a lesser extent. In Table 2.2, for example, people who have a living donor transplant in Belfast or at Guy's in London seem to have a better chance that their kidney will still be working 5 years after the operation than those who had a transplant in Leeds. There could be a number of reasons for this difference. The transplant centre in Belfast may have very strict criteria for the types of people accepted for a living donor transplant, whereas the centre in Leeds may be prepared to transplant patients who are less fit or who have other problems that might affect the success of their transplant.

It should be pointed out, however, that the BTS does not regard these results as statistically significant (i.e. they may have more to do with arbitrary differences in the populations these hospitals serve than in the standard of care provided).

Kidney Transplants Explained

Table 2.1 Survival rates for deceased donor kidneys, by centre

	1 year deceased donor graft survival	5 year deceased donor graft survival
Bristol	94	89
Coventry	95	88
St George's, London	94	87
West London	95	85
Oxford	94	85
Bart's, London	93	84
Birmingham	93	84
Cardiff	90	84
Guy's, London	92	83
Newcastle	91	82
UK average	**92**	**81**
Edinburgh	91	81
Sheffield	90	81
Nottingham	86	81
Portsmouth	89	80
Cambridge	92	79
Glasgow	91	79
Liverpool	90	79
Manchester	93	78
Leicester	90	78
Royal Free, London	89	78
Leeds	92	77
Belfast	91	75
Plymouth	90	71

The figures in this table and Table 2.2 were put together by UK transplant using records from all the transplant centres in the UK. The table shows how many transplants were still working after the first year from all those performed during 2001 to 2005. It also shows how many were still working after 5 years that were performed during 1997–2001.

The statisticians at UK transplant don't think that the figures show big differences in the performance of the transplant units, and the results shown here could have happened by chance.

Table 2.2 Survival rates for living donor kidneys, by centre

	1 year living donor graft survival	*5 years living donor graft survival*
Belfast	95	100
Guy's, London	97	95
Bristol	97	93
Leeds	97	92
Cambridge	96	92
Newcastle	96	92
West London	94	91
Birmingham	93	91
Oxford	96	90
Nottingham	94	90
Coventry	97	89
Portsmouth	94	89
UK average	**95**	**88**
St George's, London	91	87
Liverpool	90	87
Sheffield	90	87
Glasgow	97	86
Edinburgh	97	85
Leicester	97	85
Bart's, London	93	85
Cardiff	92	85
Royal Free, London	90	81
Manchester	96	79
Plymouth	75	64

NEW KIDNEYS AND OLD DISEASES

Patients who are having kidney transplants sometimes worry that the original cause of their kidney failure might make the new kidney fail too. However it is unusual for a transplanted kidney to fail from the same disease as caused the patient's original kidney failure.

An exception to this is where the original kidneys failed because the patient had a condition called focal and segmental glomerulosclerosis (FSGS). This is a type of kidney inflammation or 'glomerulonephritis', and it comes back in some, but not all, patients who have had it before. People who have lost one kidney transplant due to FSGS have a 50% chance of losing another one. There are a few other types of glomerulonephritis (including IgA nephropathy) that may also come back and affect the transplanted kidney. But these conditions, if they do recur, do not necessarily lead to loss of the kidney.

HOW DOES WHERE A KIDNEY COMES FROM AFFECT HOW LONG IT WILL WORK?

When doctors measure transplant survival, they consider two things: whether the transplant is still working (often called graft survival), and whether the patient is still alive (called patient survival). Evidence from the UK shows that people who have a living donor transplant will live longer than those receiving deceased donor transplants – having a 98% chance of being alive one year after the transplant operation, 95% chance of being alive 5 years after and 89% chance at 10 years, if the transplant is still working. This compares to a survival chance of 96%, 87% and 67% for a patient with a deceased donor transplant at the same time points.

So some doctors feel that a living donor transplant is better, as it will make you live longer. Other doctors disagree, on the grounds that this is not a fair comparison. In the past, people who received kidneys for transplant from living donors were usually younger and fitter than people who received deceased donor kidneys, although this is less likely to be the case under the new system of allocating kidneys. Also, kidneys from a living donor will, by definition, be 'fresher' as they come straight out of a living person, rather than being stored for 12–24 hours in ice-packs after being removed from a dead person.

The life expectancy of the person who has donated the kidney appears to be unaffected.

If FSGS, or one of these other conditions, were to recur in two consecutive kidneys (causing their failure) doctors would be unlikely to recommend a third transplant. If you are affected by any of these problems, you should talk to your doctor about the likelihood of the original disease recurring, and damaging a transplanted kidney.

Severe damage from diabetes recurs very rarely in a transplanted kidney, and then only after a number of years. Less than 1 in 10 kidney transplants in people with diabetes fails because of the diabetes. In addition, if a person with diabetes is able to have a pancreas transplant, their chances of diabetes-related damage to a transplanted kidney reduces even further.

Some other kidney conditions can recur in the transplanted kidney, though without always causing any damage. These include IgA nephropathy and systemic lupus erythematosus (SLE). If someone has one of these conditions, they do not need to be treated with different drugs from other transplant patients but should, like anyone with a transplant, make sure their blood pressure is carefully controlled. A check on the amount of protein in the urine every so often could provide an early warning sign of any problems.

KEY FACTS

1. Kidneys used for transplants are 'matched' to the patient's blood group and tissue type.

2. Matching the kidney to the patient lowers the risk of the body's natural defence system rejecting the kidney.

3. Everyone is born with their own blood group and tissue type and this cannot be changed.

4. In theory, the better the 'match' the higher the chances that the kidney will work.

5. In practice, matching is more important if the kidney has been out of the donor ('on-ice') for a long time.

6. Not all renal units perform kidney transplants. The renal units that don't perform transplants 'on-site' can refer their patients to any transplant centre.

3
Deceased donor transplants

This chapter describes the issues surrounding the use of kidneys from deceased donors for transplantation. We look at the different types of deceased donor, the waiting list for a deceased donor transplant and what needs to happen before you go on it. Then we look at your rights and those of the donor's family. We also provide information on preparation for the transplant operation and what to expect afterwards.

Deceased donor transplants use the kidneys that have been removed from someone who has died; approximately 65% of the kidneys transplanted in the UK come from this source. Kidneys may be removed from people who have died and are either 'heartbeating donors', or 'non-heartbeating donors'. The remaining 35% of kidneys transplanted are from living donors (see Chapter 4) (data: UKT). The proportion of transplants using kidneys from living donors is increasing each year. This is partly because fewer and fewer kidneys are available from deceased donors. But the fact that more transplants are coming from living donors is actually a good thing; as these types of transplants are easier to plan and are much more likely to be done before the patient needs to start dialysis.

HEARTBEATING DONORS

A heartbeating donor is someone who has been on a life support machine (ventilator) in an intensive care unit. They may have been killed in a car accident or have died from a stroke. The ventilator is breathing for them. Kidneys are only removed after a person has been diagnosed 'brain dead'. This means the part of the brain called the brainstem, which controls breathing, has stopped working permanently, and the person is legally certified as dead. The doctors then record this in the medical notes.

The concept of 'brain death' was developed in the 1960s when it became possible to keep brain dead patients alive almost indefinitely on ventilator machines, despite there being very little chance that they would recover. Therefore, a series of tests were developed that check the function of the brain stem and can diagnose brainstem death. These have to be performed twice by senior doctors before death can be certified. If the person who is having the brainstem death tests is considered a potential donor, their family will be approached by the intensive care team and a transplant coordinator so that possible donation of their loved one's organs can be discussed. This is obviously an enormously difficult time for the family, and all the members of the healthcare team make great efforts to support and inform the family through this period.

Research that has looked into the feelings of the families of donors has shown their grief is mostly about the death of their loved one. Organ donation cannot make this worse; in fact often the donor family sees it as a positive factor in an otherwise tragic event.

Brainstem death is irreversible, and the person's ability to breathe for him or herself will never return. A person who is brain dead will never wake up, indeed they are not only 'brain dead', but are dead. A death certificate can be issued.

If the person on the life support machine had no organs suitable for donation, the machine would be switched off at this point. If the person is going to be a donor, however, any organs for donation (such as kidneys, liver or heart) will be removed in the operating theatre. These donors are sometimes called 'heartbeating donors' as the heart is still beating when the operation starts.

As most people have two kidneys, two kidney patients are usually able to benefit from the donation of kidneys from one deceased donor.

NON-HEARTBEATING DONORS

Transplant kidneys can also be removed from people who have been dead for up to 30 minutes. These donors are called non-heartbeating (or asystolic) donors or donors after cardiac death. They may be people who have died very suddenly, usually from a heart attack, severe stroke or head injury, and have no chance of survival. Their hearts have stopped beating, and they are dead. However, they have not necessarily been put on a life support machine.

If you are given a transplant kidney from a non-heartbeating donor, it is likely that the kidney won't work straight away and you will need to have dialysis for a few days or weeks after the operation. Even if the kidney doesn't work straight away, it is just as likely to work in the long term as any other kidney from a deceased donor, and the long-term success of these transplants appears to be the same.

If you are offered a deceased donor transplant, you can ask whether it is from a heartbeating or non-heartbeating donor. You have a right to this information.

Approximately 10% of kidney transplants in the UK are from non-heartbeating donors. Most kidney transplant units in the UK now perform some transplants using kidneys from non-heartbeating donors, and would like to increase the numbers of these transplants. It is harder to organise a non-heart beating transplant than a heartbeating one, as you have to get a surgical team to the donor in less than 30 minutes. We believe that all units should make more effort to carry out such transplants. And, until they do, good kidneys are going to waste.

THE TRANSPLANT LIST

At present, not enough kidneys are donated from deceased donors to meet the demand for kidney transplants. The introduction of seat-belt laws and improvements in medicine mean that fewer people now die as a result of the accidents or illnesses that, in the past, would have made them suitable donors.

People who are waiting for a deceased donor kidney are therefore put on to a list. Their details, including their blood group and tissue type (see Chapter 2), are put onto a national computer at UK Transplant (UKT) in Bristol. When surgeons remove two kidneys from a patient who has died, UKT finds the most suitable patient for each kidney – either locally or in the rest of the country. Kidneys from heartbeating donors are allocated through this national scheme, while kidneys from non-heartbeating donors are allocated by the local transplant centre.

The national organ allocation scheme works on the basis of finding the 'right' kidney patient for the 'right' donor kidney, when one becomes available. It does not work on a 'first-come, first-served' basis. It is not really a waiting list, more of a register. A nationally agreed priority order and 'scoring system' decides where the kidneys go. Transplants are allocated to the patient who has the highest priority and points score. Points are allocated according to the best match for the kidney in terms of blood group and tissue type, and the length of time that someone has been waiting. More points are given to younger than older adults, and children have priority for well-matched kidneys. In other words, you are not joining a queue, knowing that your name will come up after a reasonably fixed period of time. However, the longer you wait, the more the points scored, and the greater the chances that you will be offered a kidney. It is important to stress though that the offer of a kidney is never guaranteed until it actually happens. There are simply not enough kidneys available to offer a transplant to everyone who is suitable.

Even though attempts have always been made to make the kidney allocation system as fair as possible, there has been a tendency for some people to be disadvantaged. This includes people with rare tissue types, who are often of Asian, black or mixed race. This disadvantage is made worse by the high number of Asian people with blood group B, because there are very few blood group B donors. Most donors are white, and their tissue type is generally more likely to be a good match for white patients. Under the kidney allocation system used in the UK in the 1990s, Asian people on the transplant list had only a 50% chance of getting a transplant compared with white people. The kidney allocation system introduced by UK Transplant in 2006 tries to make the allocation system fairer by transferring some blood group O kidneys to blood group B patients, and by making tissue typing match less important in the allocation system. However, it may still be difficult for people with an unusual tissue type to receive a transplant.

KIDNEY ALLOCATION

The way kidneys from deceased donors are allocated to people on the transplant list has changed in the last few years in the UK, but remains a topic of much debate.

The 2006 allocation system gives priority to children and young adults, those who have been waiting for a long time, and to good tissue type matching between the donor and recipient. Allocation also takes some account of the ages of the donor and recipient (so that kidneys go into a recipient of a similar age to the donor), and the distance between the donor and potential recipient (so the transplant operation can be done as soon as possible after removing the kidney from the donor). This is a national system, and a computer allocates kidneys by calculating the number of 'points' for each potential recipient.

Some people feel that this system is very inflexible. They argue especially that not everyone on the transplant waiting list is medically the same. Some people are very stable on dialysis, others have complications from dialysis and argue they will die soon if they do not receive an urgent transplant; for example, they are running out of 'access' into their bloodstream for dialysis.

The previous allocation system allowed far more kidneys to be allocated according to the unit's preference, so that 'clinical urgency' could be taken into account. Using the 2006 allocation system, about one kidney in every seven is still allocated according to centre choice, and the option of allocating kidneys to patients where the situation is clinically urgent still remains.

The current system may also be a problem for people with many antibodies against other people's tissue types, as a kidney to which they have no antibodies may be offered to someone else.

Other people say that only about 1 in 5 people on the transplant list will get a transplant every year, and that it is almost impossible to decide what is fair allocation. Why should people doing 'badly' on dialysis get priority for kidney offers? Aren't the people doing 'well' on dialysis just as deserving? Also, very few people die just because they are having problems with dialysis; they tend to have other life-threatening problems as well.

Some people think that it is up to people from ethnic minority groups to donate more organs, because at the moment more kidneys are donated by white people. However, transplant rates have increased substantially in ethnic minority patients under the new allocation scheme introduced in 2006.

The allocation system does not take account of whether people have young children to look after, or whether they will have a job and can be useful to society after a transplant. This is a concern for some people, but others say that you cannot make judgements of 'social worth' and use them to allocate healthcare treatments.

Many kidneys used to be allocated to the kidney patients who lived in the same region as the donor. This meant that patients living in parts of the country with higher donor rates and lower kidney failure rates could be four times more likely to receive a kidney than someone living in an area where there were fewer donors and more kidney patients. Some people even went so far as to move house so they could be in a 'better' donor area. However, as kidneys have become allocated on a more national basis, allocation is fairer and you should not lose out because there are fewer donors near where you live. But, as we go to press, the system has only just stopped being unfair in the way that is shown in the table on page 28.

Allocation of kidneys for transplantation is a subject that is hotly debated by UK Transplant at regular intervals. The kidney allocation system is subject to regular review, and details of the current policy are on the UK Transplant website. What do you think? The views of kidney patients are given to UK Transplant directly through patient representatives on their decision-making groups, and through local Kidney Patient Associations and the National Kidney Federation. So if you have strong views, you can – and should – make them heard.

AVERAGE WAITING TIME FOR A DECEASED DONOR KIDNEY

Measuring how long it takes to get a kidney transplant can be very difficult. This is because there are two ways of looking at the waiting times. We can either measure the average length of time that people who receive a transplant have been waiting on the list. Or we can measure the average length of time that everyone who is currently waiting for a transplant has been waiting.

The average time that people who receive a transplant have waited is nearly 2 years 6 months – currently 902 days (data: UKT). It is important to note that this is an average: it can be two days, or 20 years – or never. Worryingly, as shown in Table 3.1, there is a huge variation around the country, from 399 (just over a year) in Newcastle, to 1905 days (over five years) in Leicester. It is very difficult to say how long people have to wait for a kidney transplant. This table shows how long people who have received a transplant have had to wait.

The first column of the table shows the percentage of patients on the transplant waiting list who were transplanted within 2 years. The second column shows the number of days, on average, that people in UK renal units stay on the transplant waiting list. This table doesn't take account all of the people on the transplant waiting list who have not yet had a transplant.

As you can see, about half of people who are on the waiting list for a kidney transplant in Newcastle, Oxford, Leeds and Plymouth will receive a transplant within 2 years of going onto the transplant waiting list. This might be because these centres have more donors or less strict criteria for the patients that they accept onto the transplant waiting list. It could also be because these units have the resources to perform more transplants. Again, the 2006 changes to the allocation system should start to iron out these differences.

Apart from where you live, there are a number of other factors that may affect how long you wait. For example, if your blood group is A and you are of Caucasian (or white European) origin, you are more likely to wait less time for a kidney than if your blood group is B and you are of Asian, Chinese or Afro-Caribbean descent. This is because there are more people (and therefore more potential donors) in the UK who are of Caucasian descent, and who have blood group A, than there are people with tissue types more commonly associated with other ethnic groups. Blood group is B is the most common blood group for people of Asian descent, but B is not a particularly common blood group in the population as a whole.

Table 3.1 Time patients wait for deceased donor transplant kidneys, by centre

	Patients transplanted within 2 years (%)	Days on waiting list
Newcastle	59	399
St George's	48	545
Portsmouth	50	578
Oxford	52	599
Leeds	52	618
Cardiff	46	643
Plymouth	52	662
Guy's, London	42	719
Manchester	44	789
Liverpool	40	807
Bristol	45	825
Cambridge	41	876
UK average		**902**
Royal Free, London	32	1078
Coventry	33	1118
Bart's, London	33	1178
Glasgow	33	1179
West London	27	1281
Belfast	20	1289
Nottingham	24	1391
Birmingham	31	1512
Edinburgh	19	1693
Sheffield	21	1699
Leicester	24	1905

These figures were put together by UK transplant using records from all
the transplant centres in the UK. The way that kidneys are allocated for
transplantation changed in 2006. As a result, it is thought that the system
is now much more fair, and the differences shown in this table are improving.

There are currently about 6,500 people on the waiting list for a kidney
transplant and on average about 1,400 deceased donor kidney
transplants are performed each year. This means that 20% of the people
who are waiting on the list will get a transplant each year. At the moment

there is no record of how long all the people who haven't yet received a transplant have been waiting.

BEING ON THE TRANSPLANT LIST

There are two levels of status on the transplant list – active or suspended. Active status means that a suitable kidney may be offered. Suspended status means that a transplant will not be offered at present; though at some point, you have to be (or be likely to be) suitable for a kidney. People may be suspended from the transplant list if they go away on holiday or have an illness that makes them unfit for a transplant for a period of time. Being suspended from the transplant list does not automatically happen every time you go away on holiday. It depends how far away you are travelling. For example, if you are holidaying within the UK and could get back to your renal unit within, say 4–5 hours, you may not need to be suspended from the list. If someone is suspended, it only takes a telephone call to reactivate him or her onto the transplant list. It is important that people on the list know what their status is, to avoid being suspended by mistake. They also need to know whether they are on the list, so they know that they may be called for a transplant at any time. If you need to be suspended from the transplant list temporarily, it's up to you to tell your renal unit; and also to let them know when you are available to go back on the list.

Everyone's fitness for transplant is reviewed by his or her doctor regularly. It may sometimes be necessary to take a patient off the transplant list permanently. This may be done, for example, if someone develops a heart problem, cancer or other long-term illness. This decision would not be made lightly. Any patient whose name is removed from the list should be told about the decision. In some situations people who have been free from cancer for 5 years (though this will depend on what type of cancer it is), or who make a good recovery from a long illness, can go back onto the transplant list.

Patients who are unsure whether or not they are 'on the list' should ask their kidney doctor or nurse. They can also ask their unit staff to inform them if their name is ever taken off the waiting list. It is always worth checking that you are on the list – ask to see the information on your doctor's computer. Though even this is not foolproof. If in doubt, ask your transplant coordinator to ring UKT at Bristol. Mistakes have been made when everyone (including the doctors) *think* the patient is on the list, or has been put back onto it after a suspension – but it is a good idea to check for certain. If you have access to Renal Patient View through your hospital

---

GARY: ON THE LIST OR NOT?

Gary is 28 years old, unemployed, lives alone and has been a heroin addict. He has been free from using drugs for four years now. He has been on automated peritoneal dialysis (APD) for three years and is coping well. His doctors told him, when he started dialysis, that he was being considered for a transplant. He has few close friends and is no longer in touch with his family. No one has offered to donate a kidney to him.

As Gary has been coping well with dialysis in addition to managing to remain free from drugs for so long, he presumed that he would be on the list for transplant. He hasn't actually spoken to any of his doctors about a transplant, and was unaware that he needed to have any tests or medical assessment before going on the list.

In fact, as he had been a drug user in the past, the medical and nursing staff had assumed that he was still taking intravenous drugs. They had not considered him for a transplant, believing that he would be 'unreliable' about his treatment and might have a blood-borne infection such as hepatitis B or C. He has never been referred for the tests and isn't on the list.

Gary has shown great self-discipline in combatting his addiction. He does not have an infection, is reasonably fit and well and there may be no reason for him to be refused a transplant.

If you are not sure whether you are on the list for a transplant, you should ask. If you are in any doubt at all, check.

(see Appendix 2) then you can check your status on the transplant list yourself.

If someone is on the national transplant waiting list for a deceased donor kidney, they can still ask a relative, partner or friend to give them a kidney. Living related transplants are described more fully in Chapter 5.

DO YOU HAVE TO BE ON DIALYSIS FIRST?

Some kidney units will not put patients onto the national list for a transplant kidney until they are stable on dialysis. This is because they think it is fairer for patients from different units to start off on the transplant waiting list at the same time point in their kidney disease. However, others will put patients onto the list before they need dialysis, usually 6 months or a year before dialysis is anticipated. At this point, a person's creatinine level is likely to be about 400 µmol/L (micromoles per litre of blood); i.e. the later stages of CKD 4 with an eGFR of about 20. There is no value in going onto the transplant list years before dialysis is needed as people can usually live well with the remaining function from their own kidneys.

In 2005–6 about one in eight adult patients received a kidney transplant 'pre-emptively' – i.e. they were done before the patient needed to start dialysis. A quarter (or one in four) of adult patients having a living donor transplant were pre-emptive, and 8% (one in 12) of deceased donor kidney transplant were pre-emptive. The figures are higher for children needing transplants. About 35% (one in three) of children who received a living donor transplant did so before they needed dialysis in 2005–6 and 25% (one in four) of those who received a kidney from a deceased donor did so without going onto dialysis.

Even though kidney transplants are often effective for many years, they don't last forever. If you already have a transplant that is starting to fail, you could have a living or even a deceased donor transplant before you need to return to dialysis. If your transplant is starting to fail, do not leave discussing the issue of another transplant until the last minute. Even though it is very hard to feel you are 'giving up' on a transplant that has looked after you for years, make sure the possibility of a living transplant is addressed, and that you go on the transplant list at the right time. Just as for someone coming up to their first transplant, someone with a failing transplant would ideally have another living donor transplant just before the existing transplant fails, or go on the transplant list about 6 months before the expected time to restart dialysis.

TESTS BEFORE THE OPERATION

Even if you are called in to hospital for a transplant, this is not a guarantee you are going to receive one. Before the operation can go ahead, the doctors will need to check that you are well enough to have the operation, and that your body is unlikely to reject the transplant kidney available.

PHYSICAL EXAMINATION

First of all, the doctor will give you a thorough physical examination. The purpose of this is to check that it is safe for you to proceed with the operation. For example, if you happen to have a heavy cold on the day, you may be at risk from the anaesthetic. If you 'fail' this assessment, you will be sent home, and put back on the waiting list.

ORGANISING A TRANSPLANT BEFORE DIALYSIS IS STARTED

Some well-organised renal units are able to plan deceased donor transplants for their patients before they need dialysis. Given that it is possible, you may wonder why all hospitals don't do this. The reason is that most doctors think that because there is such a shortage of kidneys for transplantation, it is better if patients all around the UK start waiting for a kidney at an equivalent time point, i.e. when they start dialysis. This makes it fair for everyone. There are also wide variations across the UK in the time that it takes to get onto the transplant waiting list. This is because in some hospitals there can be a long delay in getting the required investigations or even an appointment to see the transplant surgeon.

Some kidney transplant centres have access to the right resources and believe that it is best to transplant patients before dialysis wherever possible. So some units do carry out more transplants before dialysis. Some transplant centres also make more effort to obtain kidneys than others and do more transplants, and some units are keener on living donor transplants than others. There are also a number of renal units that do not have a transplant centre, but who can refer their patients to more than one transplant centre in the UK, therefore getting the most out of the available opportunities for their patients. For all these reasons, patients in some units may wait less time for a transplant, be more likely to have a transplant from a living donor, and be more likely to have a transplant before they need dialysis, than is usual in other units.

THE CROSS-MATCH

This test is the final hurdle before the operation. The cross-match is a blood test to check that you have no antibodies (substances that normally help the body to fight infection) that would react against the donor kidney. High levels of such antibodies in your blood mean that the new kidney is likely to be rejected as soon as it is put into your body, even if it seems to be a good match.

What happens during a cross-match is described in Chapter 2.

BEING READY FOR A TRANSPLANT

Patients who are on the list for a transplant will not be given very much notice that a kidney is available for them. So they need to be prepared to go to the hospital at short notice. Some patients are given a 'bleep' so that they can be contacted more easily.

If you are on the transplant waiting list, it is largely up to you to ensure you can be contacted at all times, day and night. Make sure you keep your mobile phone charged, and leave it on 24 hours a day. If a kidney becomes available and you cannot be traced, it will be offered to someone else. If you take a holiday outside the UK, you should tell your hospital so that you can be suspended from the list while you are away. If you have had haemodialysis in another country, you must inform the transplant centre. This is because you may need to be screened for viruses such as hepatitis and HIV after having dialysis in some parts of the world. If you do need to be screened you will be taken off the transplant waiting list temporarily – usually for 3 months after your return from abroad.

You should be put back onto the transplant list as soon as possible after your return. You can check this has actually happened by asking your doctor to show you the computer screen or, if you have access to Renal Patient View (see Appendix 2), you can look your entry up yourself. If you are still unsure, ask your transplant coordinator to ring UKT at Bristol.

TIM: JUST IN TIME

Tim is a 24-year-old project manager for a small construction company in London. He has been on APD for 18 months, and this has fitted it in well with his lifestyle.

One weekend Tim and his girlfriend Amy travel back to their university city of Leeds for a reunion party. They plan to sleep over at a friend's house and travel back to London on Sunday. Tim accidentally leaves his mobile telephone in the car whilst he is at the party. Fortunately he remembers to retrieve it before going to bed and notices that he has had five missed calls from the hospital. He calls immediately and discovers that a kidney has become available that is a good match for him.

Amy is able to drive them back to London straight away. Tim finally arrives at the hospital in the early hours of the morning and is prepared for the operation. The staff at the transplant centre tell Tim that they were about to call another patient and offer the kidney to her. He had got in touch with them just in time.

If you 'get the call', you should go to the hospital at once. Don't have anything to eat or drink, in preparation for the anaesthetic. Drive slowly and carefully. It is better to get there five minutes 'late' than have an accident on the way.

YOU AND YOUR DONOR

Normally, if you have an operation, you have a right to be told about all the details of the surgery. This is not the case for a transplant operation, however. The guidance from the Department of Health and professional bodies is quite clear: when a transplant organ is from a deceased donor, confidentiality and feelings of the donor family have priority over the rights of the person receiving the kidney. This does not mean that there is complete secrecy, and transplant teams are sensitive and flexible in their dealings with donor families and transplant recipients.

What you will be told

You can be told the tissue match between yourself and the kidney being offered. The tissue match is described elsewhere, but you can be told whether you have a '6 out of 6', or '3 out of 6' or whatever match with the kidney.

You can ask whether the kidney is from a heartbeating or non-heartbeating donor (see pages 22–3). You have a right to know this.

You can ask if there are any problems with the kidney. For example, if there was any accidental surgical damage during retrieval, or if the kidney has been out of the donor and in ice for a long time. Generally, the longer the kidney has been out of the donor the less chance it has of working well. However, a transplant has a good chance of working even if it has been on ice for 36 hours.

You can ask if there were any medical problems with the donor that would affect the survival of the kidney. For example, sometimes doctors will take kidneys from a donor who has partial kidney failure, or is receiving temporary dialysis. It is safe to take kidneys from people with most types of brain tumour, but for some brain tumours there is a risk of the recipient getting a brain tumour some years after the transplant. There is a European Directive requiring potential recipients to be told of the risks if kidneys are taken from a donor with these types of brain tumour. As far as other types of cancer are concerned, where there is a high risk of the cancer coming back in the recipient, doctors will not take the organs and will not offer the kidneys to anyone. There is an exception to this rule, however. People who have been waiting for 15 years or more for a transplant can be offered a kidney from a donor who has had a form of cancer that is likely to come back in the recipient. As long as the doctors feel that the patient has been fully informed and is aware of the risks, such a transplant may go ahead.

SHOULD YOU ACCEPT THE KIDNEY?

As so much effort is made to find you the right kidney, you may be surprised to read that we are asking this question. But, should you? Usually, the answer is 'yes', without hesitation. But, in certain circumstances, it may be better to pause for an hour or two, and think about it. For example, if you are young, and are not yet on dialysis, you might want to consider rejecting a less well-matched kidney, or one from a donor with a brain tumour. You might be better off waiting a year or so more, for a 'better' kidney. Conversely, if you are older, and have been on dialysis for 5 years, and are running out of dialysis 'access', you might want to accept it. Part of the job of the transplant coordinator, transplant surgeon and on call kidney consultant is to advise you. Why not ask to go in and talk to them before you say 'yes', if you are not sure. Delaying the operation an hour or two will not make a huge difference.

What you will not be told

The transplant team will not tell you the name or age or ethnic origin of the donor, or where they lived. The cause of death will not be given if it might allow the recipient to guess any information about the donor, or might be upsetting to the recipient. For example, some donors have died in very tragic circumstances and it might be possible to identify the donor from newspaper reports, if even general information were given to the recipient.

Feelings in the donor family

Asking a family for permission to use organs from someone close to them who has just died will be handled sensitively by transplant coordinators. These people are specialists who are trained in this area. It is important to realise that the issue of transplantation cannot make people feel worse than they do already. In many cases the donor will have put their name onto the national Organ Donor Register at some time in the past. Using their organs for transplantation therefore respects their wishes. Under the Human Transplant Act 2006, family permission is required *only* if the wishes of the deceased are not known. If the donor's wishes about organ donation are known (whether through the Organ Donor Register or by some other means), these should take precedence over family objections. 'Lack of objection' forms are no longer used.

The use of organs for transplantation can often be a source of great consolation to a family, allowing them to feel that something good has come out of a bad situation.

Feelings in the transplant recipient

Sometimes transplant recipients feel guilty about taking a kidney from someone who has died. This is understandable, but it is important to realise that transplantation has not caused a death. On the contrary, it is one good thing that can come out of a tragic circumstance. Receiving an organ from someone who has died is not merely looking after yourself, it is providing the donor family with consolation.

If you want to talk about your feelings on this subject, do contact your local medical team, nurses or transplant coordinators, who are happy to talk and explore areas of concern. However desperately someone wants to get off dialysis and have a transplant, they still have caring feelings for others, and particularly for the families of any kidney donors. Good professional counselling is essential at this stage. Don't feel shy about asking for it as your transplant unit should be able to put you in touch with someone who can help.

SARAH AND ANNA: LOSS AND HOPE

Sarah was 30 years old, drank four cans of strong lager a day, and had done so since she left school. She worked as a clerk, and was single. Despite people, especially her sister Anna, telling her that she drank too much, she didn't think she had a problem. Then, over a period of a week, Sarah became tired, sick and stopped eating. When she became yellow in colour, she went to her local hospital where she went into liver failure rapidly, and was put on a ventilator on ITU. Despite all the efforts of the doctors, she had a brain haemorrhage and became brain dead.

Anna, her next-of-kin, gave the doctors permission to use all of Sarah's organs, except her eyes. She was later told that the two kidneys got two people off dialysis, and that her lungs and heart had saved the lives of three others. Anna often thought about these five people and occasionally wanted to meet them to 'see' a bit of Sarah. She knew it was unlikely she would get to meet them though. The transplant coordinators passed on letters from the five families to Anna. She keeps them in a box by her bed. Anna misses Sarah every day, but does find it consoling that her death has helped other people. At times she wonders if Sarah 'lives on' inside other people, but knows that this is not really the case. She has died, but she has also given new hope to other people.

CONTACTING THE DONOR FAMILY
AFTER TRANSPLANTATION

The donor family receives follow up and any counselling required from the transplant coordinators. They will receive a letter of thanks from the hospital, in which a brief comment will be made on which organs have been transplanted and how the recipients are doing.

Over a period of time after the transplant, many recipients are keen to express their gratitude to the donor family, and the transplant coordinators will act as 'go-betweens' for this type of contact.

The transplant coordinators may occasionally say that the donor family will not want any contact with the recipient, but are just satisfied with the knowledge that transplantation has taken place. In many cases, though, they will help to send a short letter of thanks, or a Christmas card, from the recipient to the donor family. Maintaining confidentiality is a priority – the coordinators will never reveal the identity of the donor or recipient to the other without a long period of consultation. Only very rarely has it been possible for the transplant recipient and donor family to meet.

HOW LONG WILL A DECEASED DONOR TRANSPLANT LAST?

The most recent research into deceased donor kidney transplants indicate that 92% (over 18 out of 20) are working after the first year, and 83% are still working five years after the operation. See also the tables in Chapter 2. This reduces to 63% 10 years after a transplant (data: UKT).

Of course, people are not statistics. Some people are lucky: their transplant lasts a lot longer.

But what do all these percentages and fractions mean for you? In other words, if you have a deceased donor kidney transplant how long will your kidney last? Well, it is difficult to say exactly, but on average, a deceased donor transplant will last about 10 years. The difficulty is that *yours* may last 20 minutes or 20 years, or it may not work at all. But the average is 10 years. Despite all the advances in medicine over recent years, doctors have still not been able to make deceased donor transplants last a lifetime. So, if you are young, you may well need more than one transplant in your life. If a transplant fails, you can restart dialysis. Then you can consider whether or not you wish to go back on the transplant waiting list. Many patients in this situation do just that.

KEY FACTS

➊ Around two thirds (65%) of kidneys transplanted in the UK come from people who have died.

➋ Deceased donor kidneys come from two sources. The vast majority (90%) are donated by people whose heart is still beating but who are brain-dead and on a life support machine. The rest are from people whose heart has stopped beating.

➌ Kidneys from deceased donors work well: 92% are still working a year after the operation, 83% after five years, and 63% after 10 years.

➍ The transplant 'waiting list' is for patients waiting for deceased donor kidneys.

➎ Patients can go onto the transplant list as soon as they have had a 'work-up'. This could be before they have started dialysis.

➏ The waiting list has a national allocation scheme. This works on the basis of finding the 'right' (best-matched) patient in the UK for the 'right' kidney; it does not work on a 'first-come, first-served' basis.

➐ It is difficult to say exactly how long patients wait for a transplant; but people who get a transplant will wait on average 2½ years.

➑ Some patients might have to wait longer than 2½ years if a suitable kidney cannot be found. Some patients wait less time.

➒ It is possible to find out some information about a deceased donor kidney, but you will not be told the name of the donor. Some transplant patients send anonymous letters of thanks to the donor family.

4
Living donor transplants

In this chapter, we discuss the issues surrounding living donor transplantation, the procedures and processes involved, the benefits of this type of transplant, and some of the possible problems.

In the UK, the majority of kidneys for transplantation are donated by people who have died (deceased donor transplants). However, a significant proportion of kidneys (currently over 35% in the UK) are donated from another family member or someone who is close to the person with kidney failure. Human beings do not need two kidneys – quite why we have a 'spare one' is not known. But people with two healthy and well-functioning kidneys are unlikely to come to any harm if they lose or donate one of them.

A transplant from a living donor can have many benefits. For most patients, being given a transplant kidney from a living donor will be their best chance of having a transplant operation before they actually need dialysis. If someone close to them is able to donate a kidney, the whole transplant procedure can be planned well before dialysis. This means that both donor and recipient will be well at the time of operation. It can be scheduled around their life and work commitments.

However, there are risks with the procedure. Just as with a deceased donor transplant, the kidney may not work. Although 19 out of 20 living donor transplants are working a year after the transplant, that means 1 out of 20 has failed. This the most important risk of a living donor transplant. So it is worth considering the emotional aspects of living transplantation before embarking on the process. Both you and your donor need to talk about the possibility of complications following the operations, and how both of you might feel if the transplant doesn't work.

Anyone who is on the list for a deceased donor transplant can have a living donor transplant if they have a suitable donor. A growing number of transplant units now have a living donor coordinator whose main job is to organise living donor transplants. This is part of the reason why these transplants are becoming more common.

Even if you are on the deceased donor transplant waiting list, but are also having the necessary tests for a living donor transplant, you may be lucky enough to be offered a deceased donor organ. You will then have a difficult decision to make: should you, or should you not, accept the organ. This decision is made harder by the fact that living donor transplants may have better results. If the deceased donor organ is not a good match, or it is not a particularly 'good' organ, it may be better to say 'no', and proceed with the living donor transplant. On the other hand, if both you and your donor are reasonably young and fit, it may be better to take the deceased donor kidney, knowing that your living donor may be available in 10 or 20 years time (should you need another transplant). But, ultimately, the decision is a personal one for you to discuss with your family, your donor and the doctors.

WILL A LIVING DONOR TRANSPLANT LAST ANY LONGER?

Evidence from UK data is that living donor transplants last longer than deceased donor transplants – having a 95% chance of still working 1 year after the transplant operation, 89% chance of working 5 years after and 65% chance at 10 years (data: UKT). This compares with a survival chance of a deceased donor kidney of 92%, 82% and 63% at the same time points. The gap between the results is narrowing.

Although these figures seem to show some advantage from living donor transplantation, they may overestimate any advantage. Until recently, living donor kidneys tended to come from younger fitter donors, and be put into younger fitter recipients who had not been on dialysis for long (if at all). In other words, some doctors feel they cannot say that, for an individual patient, a living donor transplant is more likely to work than a deceased donor transplant. Nor can they say categorically that it is more likely to make that particular patient live longer.

WHO CAN DONATE A KIDNEY?

Almost anyone can donate a kidney to a loved one. The best donor is an identical twin, as the whole genetic make-up (including blood group and tissue type) are identical. Unfortunately, most people do not have an identical twin waiting to give them a kidney! A kidney from a non-identical twin may also be suitable, but no more so than a kidney from a brother or sister born separately. If a kidney patient has a friend, partner or relative who is at least 18 years old (16 in Scotland), healthy, and willing to give them a kidney, they should speak to the transplant coordinator (or other senior nurse or doctor) at their unit.

'First-degree' relatives (i.e. a brother, sister, father, mother, son or daughter) are likely to be particularly good as donors. Other more distant relatives may also be suitable however – particularly an uncle, aunt, nephew, niece, cousin, grandparent or grandchild. In fact, the donor does not necessarily have to be a blood relative. The patient's wife, husband, partner or close friend may also be suitable.

As human beings do not need two kidneys to be healthy, the donor is unlikely to come to any harm by losing a kidney. However, before the operation can take place, the donor must have rigorous tests to make sure that he or she is fit enough to give up a kidney.

There are some situations where it would not be possible for a living person to donate a kidney. These include people with the following conditions:

- HIV or AIDS-related infection;

- Hepatitis B or C infection;

- Creutzfeldt-Jakob disease (CJD);

- Major heart or breathing problems;

- Diabetes;

- Significant kidney disease;

- Most cancers;

- Very high blood pressure (i.e. blood pressure requiring several drugs to control, or that has caused strain to the heart or circulation);

- Intravenous drug abuse;

- Extreme obesity;

- Pregnancy (at the time or planned in the very near future);

- Having only one kidney;

- Evidence of financial or non-financial coercion;

- Inability of a potential donor to give informed consent;

- Age below 18 years (or 16 in Scotland).

In addition, doctors would think very seriously before recommending any-one to donate a kidney if any of the following applied:

- Age over 70 years;

- Intellectual impairment but able to give informed consent;

- Mild obesity;

- Family history of diabetes, or autoimmune disease (e.g. SLE, nephritis) as the donor may be more likely than average to develop such a disease in later life and these diseases can affect the kidneys;

- Any medical condition that might put the patient at risk of future kidney disease;

- Mild high blood pressure.

Who will do the asking?

It is up to kidney patients to ask their friends or family to see if they are will-ing to donate a kidney. Doctors will not usually go and ask a patient's loved ones for them, but they will talk to anybody who is willing to donate a kidney and gets in touch with them. Living donor coordinators may be able to help you decide the best approach as it can be difficult to ask. Some transplant centres will approach donors directly in writing, with the recip-ient's permission. Discussing the best way for you is very important.

TESTS BEFORE LIVING DONOR TRANSPLANTATION

Tests for the recipient are the same as those for deceased donor transplant outlined in Chapter 3.

On average, it can take up to six months to prepare for a living donor transplant. We feel that this is too long. Even though there is no national target for the work-up process, the government's new 18 week target for a 'completed outpatient episode' is a good target for transplant work-up too. This means that the time taken from deciding that a donor-recipient pair may be suitable to transplant, then (if they are suitable) to being able to do the operation, should be about four months. In an emergency situation, it may take a week, but this is very unusual. Sometimes, the time is deliber-ately long in order to give both parties sufficient time for careful consideration. The most important thing is to tailor the assessment to the needs of the donor and recipient.

The first, and perhaps the most important test that is done to see

WHO WILL MAKE THE MOST SUITABLE DONOR?

Not everyone has relatives or close friends who are in a position to donate kidneys, but some patients are lucky in this regard. A few may actually be inundated with offers of kidneys when told they will need a transplant. If you are lucky enough to have more than one potential donor, it can be difficult to decide whose kidney to accept. Each of your possible donors will be assessed for their medical suitability for donation, and to ensure they are in good health before, during and after the operation.

Some would say that if a patient has a parent and a brother, sister or partner, all of whom are willing (and able) to donate, it might be 'better' to accept the kidney from the parent now, and then 'keep' the sibling's or partner's kidney for later in life, if the first transplant ever fails. Others would say take the kidney from the younger person, as they are more likely to be fitter and get through the operation without problems. Alternatively, what if no parent is suitable, but both a brother and partner are suitable, which should you choose? There are no hard and fast rules. The situation will vary between different patients; each individual will have different relationships with the members of their family circle, and will not necessarily feel closest to their nearest blood relative. It may seem strange to think of friends and relatives in this way, but the reality of living donor transplants means that such issues need to be considered.

There is no evidence that a woman of childbearing age (provided she is not actually pregnant at the time) will be at any more risk than anyone else who is offering to be a donor. Nor is there any evidence that it will affect her chance of getting pregnant, or put a future pregnancy at risk.

whether the potential transplant might work, is a simple blood test to find out the blood group of the donor. Usually, if the patient's blood group and the donor's blood group are not compatible (according to the rules outlined on pages 12–13), no further tests will be carried out. The transplant is unlikely to go ahead, so the tests will be stopped.

Some transplant centres are now introducing a new technique called antibody incompatible transplantation (see page 59). This is making successful transplants more likely when a donor is the 'wrong' blood group. On the other hand, if you are being offered a kidney by more than one friend or relative, it would make sense to go for the one who is blood group compatible with yours first.

If the blood groups of the donor and recipient are compatible, blood samples will be taken to test the donor's liver and kidney function. If these prove satisfactory, the rest of the donor evaluation can be planned.

It is important that the donor plans for time off work before the transplant as well as after the operation. He or she is likely to need several days off, taken as single days. This is to ensure there is time to do all the necessary tests to ensure that this person is suitable to donate a kidney. Tests cause many problems for donors as they are fitted into the hospital system and there may be cancellations or delays. Each test, it would seem, is looked at individually and no attempt seems to be made to make them convenient for the donor. You can discuss this with the transplant coordinator and see if appointments can be scheduled better.

The donor will need to have a thorough medical examination. Two separate doctors usually do this – a kidney doctor (usually a different one from the doctor responsible for the patient), and the surgeon who will perform the operation. The doctors are interested in the person's general health as well as the health of their kidneys. They will check to make sure that the donor has a normal blood pressure. If his or her blood pressure is found to be high, the doctors may monitor it for 24 hours – this is because it may be high only at certain times of the day, or in certain circumstances. In some cases, the doctors may still agree to go ahead with the transplant, even if the donor has high blood pressure, just as long as it is well controlled using only one type of blood pressure tablet, and there is no evidence that the high blood pressure has put a strain on the heart or kidneys.

An ultrasound scan will then usually be used to make sure that the donor has two kidneys, and that both are functioning equally well. The function of the individual kidneys may then be measured more accurately by a test such as a nuclear medicine test. Each kidney should be providing 50% of the total kidney function. It is no good if one kidney is doing more work than the other. If the surgeon then removed the kidney that did most of the work, this could be disastrous for the donor.

The potential donor will also have an ECG (a heart trace) and a chest X-ray to ensure there are no problems with their heart or breathing. They may also be given an exercise tolerance test, to see how their heart reacts under gentle exercise, and an ECHO (echocardiogram, an ultrasound of the heart). If there is any doubt about the heart, it may be necessary to see a heart specialist. Quite a few apparently healthy people in their 40s and 50s have finished up with heart surgery or angioplasty after kidney donor screening. Over the next few years, it may be possible to check the heart of a potential donor using a CT scan, as the newer machines can take much more detailed images. This helps doctors to be sure that the donor has a healthy heart.

The donor will have blood tests to make sure they don't have infections such as HIV, hepatitis B or C, cytomegalovirus (CMV), Epstein-Barr virus (EBV) or other viruses; these may be transmitted with the transplant. It is also important to know the relationship between donor and recipient. Blood samples will also be used to test the donor's genetic compatibility (tissue type) with the recipient's. This is necessary for all live related donor transplants so that the genetic relationship between donor and recipient can be proven. Tissue-type matching is also undertaken to find out whether the donor and recipient are well matched. However, close matching is not vital in living donor transplants (see page 15 for more details).

In addition, there will also be a cross-match test (see page 13) between donor and recipient. As with deceased donor transplantation, if the cross-match is negative, this means the transplant work-up can continue. But if the cross-match is positive, the transplant cannot go ahead unless a procedure called antibody incompatible transplantation is performed (see page 59).

A psychological assessment of both donor and recipient may be carried out in some situations. This is to make sure that both are happy about the procedure, and the effects it may have on them and their families. The psychologist will make sure that both people (and their families) are able to cope if the transplant fails, or if anything happens to either of them during surgery. Access to a psychologist or counsellor should always be available.

Finally, to help the surgeons decide which kidney to remove from the donor (left or right), the blood vessels to each kidney must be examined using a scan called a computed tomography angiogram (CTA) or magnetic resonance angiogram (MRA). These scans take a special look at the blood vessels to the kidneys and are essential in planning which kidney to take out. They can also tell the surgeon whether they have to take account of variations in the numbers of blood vessels to each kidney.

RISKS TO THE DONOR

There is about a 1 in 3,000 risk of the donor dying as a result of the operation. This is similar to the risk of having almost any operation. The risks to a healthy donor should be minimal if all the pre-operative tests have been carried out.

A kidney specialist doctor should see anyone who donates a kidney regularly after the operation. UK Guidelines recommend that kidney donors should be seen at least once a year for the rest of their life. Donor follow-up is usually performed by nurses, though it may become the responsibility of the GP or a surgeon or nephrologist at your local renal unit. There is some evidence to suggest that kidney donors live longer than other people on average – nobody knows why this might be so. Although it might perhaps be that they are motivated to take good care of themselves, and are known to be fit and healthy at the time of donation.

The whole living donation process is an emotional rollercoaster ride for both the donor and recipient. Every test is a hurdle, a bit like the Grand National. You will be in constant fear of failure, and ecstatic when you 'pass'! Both donor and recipient will need a lot of help and support, and donors should make sure that they have contact with the transplant centre. If you are lucky, all the support you need will be available from a good transplant coordinator who becomes your best friend.

KEY FACTS

1. Around a third (35%) of kidneys transplanted in the UK come from people who are still alive.

2. Most healthy people (friend, partner or relative) can donate a kidney to a loved one and survive perfectly well with just one kidney.

3. Kidneys from living donors work well: 95% are still working a year after the operation, 89% after five years and 65% after 10 years.

4. Before a living donor transplant can happen, both the donor and the recipient need to have tests to make sure the operation will be successful.

5. It is less important, when compared to a deceased donor transplant, that the donor and recipient be a good 'match', in terms of tissue type and blood group.

6. Patients and donors may also have psychological tests before a living donor transplant, to make sure that they are both aware of the consequences of the procedure.

5
The donor's operation

This chapter looks at what it is like for the donor to have a kidney removed, and considers what risks are involved for a living donor.

There are two methods of surgically removing a kidney from a living donor: open surgery, or laparoscopic surgery (using keyhole surgery). The removal of a kidney is called a nephrectomy. Donors often ask if they will be given the choice of having the operation at a unit where a laparoscopic nephrectomy is available. As it is available in a small number of transplant centres only, the benefits have to be weighed against the inconvenience of having to travel long distances. Also the research shows that there is no real difference in how long it takes a person to recover from the operation, whichever method of surgery is used.

OPEN NEPHRECTOMY (OPEN SURGERY)

The surgeon makes a cut under the donor's ribcage that is about 15–20 cm long. Most surgeons take the kidney out from the front of the donor, rather than from the side, which was usual a few years ago (but very rare now). This is because part of a rib may also need to be removed if the kidney is removed from the side of the abdomen. Taking the kidney out from the front of the tummy leaves a smaller scar and causes less pain than removing it from the side, but both methods leave a longer scar than keyhole surgery. It also takes longer for the donor to recover after the operation, perhaps as much as three months to be 'back to normal'.

LAPAROSCOPIC NEPHRECTOMY (KEYHOLE SURGERY)

Some kidney transplant surgeons remove kidneys from living donors using keyhole surgery. A small cut is made above the pubic hairline (a 'bikini' or 'low bikini' cut). During the operation, a laparoscope (a tiny camera on the end of a long cable) is inserted into the tummy. In fact, three of these are used – two inserted from the side and one near the tummy button. The surgeon uses the cameras to locate the kidney and then it can be removed

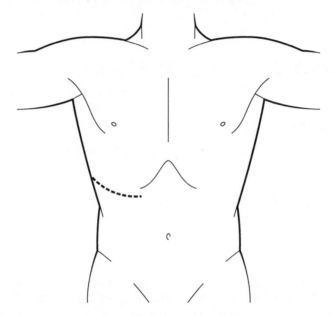

Figure 5.1 Open nephrectomy

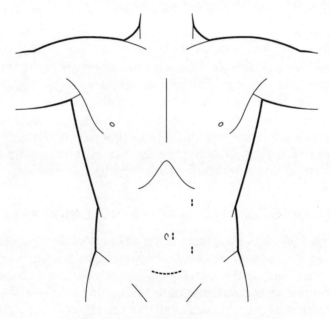

Figure 5.2 Laparascopic nephrectomy

through a cut about 15cm long, made 5 cm below the tummy button (along the 'bikini line'). Some surgeons use this cut to feed their hand into the tummy, so that they do the operation partly with the keyhole surgical instruments and partly with their hand. Other surgeons do the whole operation using keyhole instruments. Although surgeons can spend hours discussing the merits of each approach, there are no proven differences in the safety or outcomes of these two techniques.

If there is a problem during the operation, the surgeon may have to change to an open procedure. If they don't, the donor should recover in four weeks, or less.

The operation to remove a kidney for live donation usually takes between one and a half and two and a half hours. It is important to remember that the time in between leaving the ward and returning is much longer. It takes time to put someone to sleep before the operation, and people remain under observation in a recovery room for a while after the operation so that the anaesthetist can check they have woken up fully. This is something over which your hospital team will take great care.

LAPAROSCOPIC NEPHRECTOMY vs NEPHRECTOMY

If a kidney is removed from the donor using conventional 'open surgery', there is significantly less risk that the donated kidney will be damaged during the operation to remove it, though laparoscopic nephrectomy does have benefits. The donor will have a smaller scar and is likely to recover more quickly than donors whose kidney is removed by open surgery. However there are some disadvantages to laparoscopic nephrectomy. It takes time for transplant surgeons to learn how to perform the laparoscopic operation. It is also important for the surgeon to perform the operation regularly to keep in practice. This may not be possible in some UK transplant centres where living donor transplants are not performed very often. It is a good idea to ask your surgeon how many laparoscopic nephrectomies he or she has done before. More than 100, including several recent ones, should give you confidence that the operation will be safe. If the surgeon is learning the technique, he or she will be closely supervised by an expert. So you should also ask these questions about the consultant in charge.

Whichever method is used to remove a kidney for live donation, the surgeon always takes great care not to damage the organ in any way. The surgeon also removes the blood vessels and a short length of the tube (ureter) that drains the urine towards the bladder, as they will be used for the recipient.

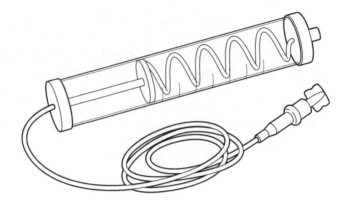

Figure 5.3 A PCA pump

AFTER THE OPERATION

After the operation, the donor will have a drip in the arm to give fluids, and a catheter tube into the bladder so that the urine from the remaining kidney can be measured. Painkillers will be given; it is best to check with the surgeon before the operation how this will be done. It is common practice now for people who have just had surgery to have a strong painkiller given by a drip. They can control the dose of the painkiller by pressing a button on a band placed on their wrist (a 'patient controlled analgesia' or 'PCA' pump). Anyone donating a kidney should be taught how to use such a device before having the operation. To prevent an overdose of painkiller, the device will only allow a certain amount of painkiller to be given at a time. If you are still in pain despite receiving a painkiller in this way, it is important to ask the nurses or doctors for more painkillers.

Pain relief after the operation may also include an epidural anaesthetic. While this is unlikely to be needed following laparoscopic nephrectomy, it can be very helpful after open nephrectomy. It is a good idea to ask the staff caring for you if you can have this form of pain relief before you have the operation, so that staff can be prepared.

Most people who donate a kidney will experience some pain and discomfort after the operation. This usually gets better after a few days. Three months after the operation, the majority of donors will feel no pain at the operation site. However, one in 25 people who have donated a kidney by open (as opposed to laparoscopic) surgery do suffer from long-term pain at the site of the wound. A pain specialist may be able to offer treatment such as injections into the wound.

In the few days after the operation, about one out of three donors will get a minor complication of one kind or another. This might be a urine infection, or some sickness or slight delay in opening their bowels. About 1 in 10 donors will get a more serious complication such as pneumonia (a lung infection), wound infection, or a blood clot in the veins of the leg that could move to the lungs. These are complications that might affect anyone who has had an operation. They are not specific to donating a kidney.

It is important to reduce the risks of blood clots in the legs (deep vein thrombosis or DVT), since blood clots can travel to the lungs and block the blood supply ('pulmonary embolus'). Careful planning and care before the operation are important. You will have tests to make sure you are not at high risk of developing complications. Injections of a drug (heparin) that prevents clotting of the blood will be given each day. To keep the circulation in the legs moving, you are likely to be given special 'anti-embolism' stockings to wear before the operation. After the operation, you will have a good chance of avoiding complications if you do breathing exercises while in bed, and also if you sit out of bed and start to walk around as soon as possible after the operation. A physiotherapist will advise and help you with these activities.

The majority of donors have no complications, however, and leave hospital soon after the operation. If the kidney is removed using laparoscopic nephrectomy, the donor will be in hospital for about 3–5 days, but after open surgery this could be 5–9 days.

How soon the donor returns to work will depend on the type of work and the person's general level of fitness before the operation. If the work is physically demanding, the donor will probably need a longer recovery time than someone who's work is sedentary. If the kidney is donated by laparoscopic nephrectomy, the donor can probably return to work within four weeks of the operation. With open surgery, it is advisable to remain off work for about three months.

In some ways the donor has a 'bigger' operation than the recipient. Firstly, donors have a bigger wound than recipients, as their scar may cut across the lower chest and upper abdomen (see Figure 5.2 on page 48). Secondly, donors are fit and healthy before the operation, whereas recipients usually feel poorly. After the operation the recipient is likely to feel a lot better than they did before, but the donor won't. In fact, initially they will feel worse, especially as they have the anxiety of not knowing at this stage whether their kidney will work inside their loved one.

One of the biggest problems of donating a kidney to someone you care about is the potential emotional upset if the transplant fails at an early stage. Fooling yourself into believing you could cope is a real danger. If the worst *does* happen, both donor and recipient will need a great deal of support from their renal unit staff as well as from friends and family. This also applies if the kidney fails some years down the line, and particularly if someone dies.

There is usually a 10–20% rise in the donor's creatinine level after losing a kidney, reflecting a slight reduction in overall kidney function. Some donors may develop protein in their urine (proteinuria) but this is usually mild and not harmful. If there is protein in the urine, doctors will be stricter about blood pressure control and monitor it very carefully. However, if the creatinine is not continuing to rise after the first year, there is no need for any concern.

About 10% of all donors find their blood pressure goes up, so this will need to be checked regularly. They may end up needing tablets to control it. Either way you will not 'feel anything' if there is a problem with the creatinine or blood pressure; they just have to be checked.

After a living transplant, most of the focus is (inevitably) on the recipient. But actually, at this stage, it is the donor who is having the bigger operation. They may go home first, often within a week, but their follow-up has to be nearly as careful as that given to the person who now has their kidney. If they are well, they should be seen by a senior doctor, and bloods checked, at four weeks and three months; then yearly, for the rest of their lives.

It is essential, however, that living donors realise that they have not become renal patients. They are healthy people who have given a kidney so that another person can have a normal life. On the rare occasions that donors do start to see themselves as patients following a nephrectomy, they tend to develop problems of various kinds – such as health problems, relationship problems, problems with anxiety and depression.

It is also advisable for living donors to check their mortgage insurance, life insurance and credit card insurance, to ensure they are not invalidated by volunteering for the operation. The NKF and the Edinburgh Royal Infirmary transplant unit did some work in this area a few years ago. As a result, the five largest British life insurance companies agreed to accept continuity of donor cover during the transplant operation and the continuity of donor cover remains unchanged after the operation. This agreement is based on evidence presented by the NKF and REI and should still be valid, although problems may still arise from time to time. If ever you have difficulties with continuity of insurance cover, you should inform your own hospital and contact the NKF (see Appendix 2 for address).

KEY FACTS

1. The operation to remove a kidney from a living donor takes about 2 hours and has the same risks as other major surgery.

2. There are two ways in which the kidney can be removed: by open nephrectomy, or by laparoscopic nephrectomy (keyhole surgery). Laparoscopic nephrectomy is a more complicated technique but if it is performed by a competent surgeon, recovery should be considerably quicker.

3. The scar left after a laparoscopic nephrectomy is smaller than the one left by open nephrectomy.

4. Living donors spend about a week in hospital after the operation. The transplant recipient will need to stay in hospital for about 10–14 days, if there are no complications.

5. When they are well, people who donate a kidney should have check-ups every year after the operation.

6. Just because a kidney has been provided by a living donor doesn't necessarily mean that all will go well. Both patient and donor will need a lot of support if the transplant should fail, and should be offered professional counselling.

6
Living donor transplantation: some considerations

This chapters looks at the risks involved for the person receiving a kidney from a living donor, and considers some of the other ethical issues and dilemmas that can arise from living donor transplantation.

For the recipient, a living donor kidney transplant operation carries the same risks as a deceased donor transplant (see Chapter 3).

REJECTION

Unless the living donor transplant has come from an identical twin, there will be a risk of the recipient's body rejecting the kidney. Around a quarter (25%) of patients may experience rejection at some point in the first year after a transplant – however this doesn't always mean that the transplant kidney will stop working. This is about the same as the risk for people who have had a deceased donor transplant. This is why it is very important for patients to take their immunosuppressant medication exactly as it has been prescribed, to help avoid rejection. More information about rejection, other problems that can occur in the first few weeks, and immunosuppressant medication is given in the following chapters.

If a kidney that has been donated to you by someone you love fails, this can be extremely upsetting – both for you and for your donor. If this should happen, it is very important you are both put in touch with a professional counsellor who can help you deal with the feelings that are bound to arise (see also Chapter 4).

SOME ADVANTAGES OF LIVING DONOR TRANSPLANTS

Transplanted kidneys from living donors are more likely to work straight away than those from deceased donors. It is often easier to identify problems in these kidneys than it is in kidneys from deceased donors.

A kidney from a living donor is likely to function for longer than a deceased donor kidney. The latest figures from the UK show that 95% of living donor transplants were still working after the first year (that is approximately 19 out of 20), 89% were still working after 5 years and 65% after 10 years. This is in contrast to only 92% of deceased donor transplants at one year (about 18 out of 20), 83% at 5 years, and 63% after 10 years (data: UKT). Again, the gap between the results is narrowing, perhaps for the reasons suggested in Chapter 2.

These statistics are all very well, but anyone considering accepting a kidney from a living donor will want to know how long a living transplant will last for them. As with a deceased donor kidney (see Chapter 3), any individual living donor transplant may last 20 minutes or 20 years, or indeed it may not work at all. But, on average, a living donor transplant will last 15 years or more (that is 5 or more years of 'additional kidney life' when compared to a deceased donor kidney).

Even 15 years is not that long, if you go into established renal failure (ERF) at a young age. In other words, young patients may well need more than one transplant in their lives, whether or not their transplants are from living donors.

Many doctors and nurses think that if both sides are willing, and understand and accept the risks, it is 'better' for most patients to have their first transplant from a living donor. This is especially important in families, such as Asian and black families, where a suitable deceased donor kidney is likely to be harder to come by. This is because there is a shortage of kidneys donated from Asian and black people. A kidney is much more likely to be a better 'match' (see Chapter 2) if it comes from someone of a similar ethnic group.

Other people think that there is no point taking the risks of removing a kidney from a living person, when removing a kidney from a dead person will do no further harm (as they are already dead). In addition, the difference in survival of the kidney transplant and patient between living and deceased donor kidneys is very biased. Until the introduction of the allocation scheme in 2006, far more young people were receiving living donor transplants and living donors tend to be younger and fitter than deceased ones. There is some evidence that this is now starting to change, however.

Another reason for this bias is that living donors are carefully screened for any diseases that might affect their kidneys, such as hypertension or diabetes. The donor's kidneys are also checked to make sure that they function perfectly, and are not likely to fail in the future. Also, a living donor transplant is more likely to be done before dialysis is needed and therefore the recipient may also be slightly fitter than if they were on dialysis.

Also, the time in which the kidney is outside a human body after it has been removed from the donor (i.e. 'still fresh') – called the cold ischaemia time – seems to be a crucial factor. This is less than one hour for a living donor transplant, but 12–36 hours (the average is 18–20 hours) for a deceased donor transplant. The benefits of transplanting the kidney as soon as it is removed from the donor seem to be more important than other issues such as tissue type, for the success of the transplant.

In the end, you decide. It is up to each donor and recipient pair to make the decision, having taken in the type of information put forward in this chapter, and discussed this with their doctors and the rest of their family. It is not unusual for some friends or relatives to be very afraid of the risks involved in donation; whatever their reasons this must be respected. It can also happen that a donor wishes to back out, sometimes very close to the operation. Again it is essential that such events are respected and handled sympathetically to allow the donor or prospective donors to back out, without the risk of recrimination particularly from other family members. Refusal of a spouse to let their partner donate is not uncommon, even when the partner is desperate to help. Discussion and counselling can often help.

JOEL'S DILEMMA: WHICH BROTHER TO CHOOSE?

Joel is a 46-year-old man who has had kidney failure for about six years. He's been on haemodialysis since his diagnosis. He was told he needed to stop smoking and lose 2 stone in weight before he could go on the transplant list. It has taken him 18 months to achieve this. He has a close family with four brothers, and a sister. All of his siblings have offered to donate a kidney; however only two of his brothers are a good match. These brothers have always had a competitive relationship. At school they were both strong sportsmen and competed in county athletics championships. They now see the 'race' to donate a kidney as a competition and their relationship is deteriorating as a result.

Joel feels very uneasy about accepting a kidney from either of them, as he feels responsible for their quarrels. Should Joel wait for a deceased donor transplant, or should he accept a kidney from one brother, in the knowledge that he may well need his other brother's kidney later, when the first one fails?

A living donor transplant often improves the relationship between donor and recipient, as there is a common bond between the two. However, relationships can be complicated and this may not always be the case.

Living donor transplants are becoming more common in the UK, but there is still a large shortfall in the number of kidneys being offered for donation in relation to the number of people wanting a transplant. Hopefully, with better awareness of the higher success rate of living donor transplants, the number will continue to rise. Even though many nurses and doctors favour living over deceased donor transplants, it is not a simple issue and you need to weigh up the pros and cons of each approach.

WHY ARE THERE MORE LIVING DONOR TRANSPLANTS IN SOME AREAS THAN IN OTHERS?

Some renal units in the UK do not promote living donor transplantation as actively as others. This means that there is a wide variation in the rate of living donor transplants carried out, almost like a 'postcode lottery'.

The proportion of living donor transplants is increasing every year. Even though overall in the UK, 35% of transplants are living donor ones, in some UK units they now account for as many as 50% of all kidney transplant operations.

Why this is, is unclear. There may be differences in opinion between different doctors and units, in terms of the morality of living donor transplantation. Some doctors are still uncomfortable as operating on a healthy person goes against one of the most basic motives of a doctor ('do no harm').

The units with higher rates match the European 'leader' in living transplantation, Sweden, where 44% of all kidneys transplanted in 2005–6 came from living donors. In countries, such as Japan, where deceased donor transplantation is almost unheard of for cultural reasons, living transplant offers the only real option to coming off or avoiding dialysis. On the other hand, in some European countries such as France and Spain there is virtually no living donor transplantation, as it does not seem to be encouraged by doctors. Even the transplant units in the UK with lower living donor transplant rates are well above these countries. Spain compensates for this by having a high rate of deceased donor transplants. The Spanish success in finding plenty of deceased donor kidneys means that the need for living donor kidneys is reducing – but it has not disappeared entirely.

THE HUMAN TISSUE AUTHORITY (HTA)

Before any living donor transplant can go ahead, a relationship between the donor and recipient must be proved that is sufficiently strong to justify kidney donation. This relationship may be between blood relatives or an emotional relationship, for example between partners, friends or spouses.

Every donor and recipient pair must go through an independent assessment by a trained assessor who acts on behalf of a government agency called the Human Tissue Authority or HTA, to ensure that all the legal requirements are met. The assessor will see the donor in private, and check that there is no coercion or reward for donating the kidney. The HTA assessor may be a doctor, but not a kidney specialist, or another healthcare professional who is not a member of the transplant team. The report from the independent assessor to the HTA needs to be supported by evidence of a genetic relationship if there is one. If the two people involved are not genetically related, they will need to supply documentary evidence. This may include a marriage certificate, photographs of the donor and recipient together over a considerable period of time, or evidence of co-habitation.

The Human Tissue Authority produces a helpful leaflet entitled *Information about living donor transplants*. This is available in paper form or can be downloaded from the website (see Appendix 2 for address details).

The HTA's role is to ensure that the kidney is being donated freely and for no other reason than to benefit the recipient's health. The assessor makes a report to the HTA central office, which then decides whether to approve the transplant. The HTA undertakes to make the assessment within 5 working days, although collecting all the evidence may take much longer. Incomplete or incorrect evidence could slow the process and delay the HTA being able to approve.

The HTA also regulates other types of transplantation and artificial fertilisation. You can find out more about the work of the HTA from the website address given in Appendix 2.

Even though it is illegal to offer payment to enable the living donor transplant to take place, the National Health Service will repay the donor reasonable costs incurred due to travelling (even from abroad) or loss of earnings. This facility was included in the Human Organ Transplant Act (1989) and remains in the more recent Human Tissue Act. Your transplant coordinator will know how to obtain this money from the Health Authority or Primary Care Trust. A potential donor will be asked to provide evidence of three or more months' earnings (for example, payslips, accountant's tax returns). There is some variation around the country,

---

LYNNE AND SUSAN: ARE THEY CLOSE ENOUGH?

Lynne and Susan have known each other since primary school and each is godmother to one of the other's children. Lynne's kidneys failed ten months ago when she was in her mid-40s. She had to give up her job as an airline stewardess as it proved impossible to fit around her dialysis sessions. Although her husband earns enough for them to survive (he's a supermarket manager) they can no longer afford holidays or extra luxuries.

Susan wants to offer one of her kidneys to her oldest and closest friend. How do they go about amassing the proof that their relationship is a genuine one and that the offer of a kidney is because of longstanding friendship rather than for other reasons?

They decide to put together a photo album of their lives. This includes photographs from school, holidays together as teenagers, and letters that they sent while they were both at college in different parts of the country. They put in pictures of the Christenings of their children, along with copies of the baptism certificates. They are also able to include testimonies from other people – friends, relatives, and Mrs Parker who taught them both when they were 14.

They have separate interviews with the HTA assessor. Susan is keen to make it clear that she doesn't want any form of payment for the kidney and is able to show that she is financially secure, in no debt, and has an established career as an HR consultant.

Their case is accepted, and plans are made for the transplant to go ahead.

---

but most donors can receive up to three months reimbursement of earnings and some reasonable expenses. If someone has very high earnings, some Primary Care Trusts will be reluctant to reimburse fully, capping the earnings reimbursement.

ANTIBODY INCOMPATIBLE TRANSPLANTS (AIT)

Tests on the donor and patient's blood, and the cross-match test between donor and patient, may indicate that the patient has antibodies that will fight an organ from the donor. These may increase the risk of rejection, and for many years doctors would not perform a transplant in the face of damaging antibodies. Similarly, if a patient has antibodies against a kidney from a deceased donor, the transplant would be given to someone else in preference. Or the donor kidney may have the wrong blood group. This would normally make the transplant impossible

Doctors have spent many years trying to get around the problem of antibodies preventing transplantation, and/or blood group incompatibility. From about 1970 to 1995, many strategies were developed to overcome the problems, and research showed that some antibodies could be safely ignored. This, however, still left many people without transplants.

Since 1995, programmes of 'Antibody Incompatible Transplantation, AIT' (also called densensitisation) have become more successful; and everyone in the UK should either have a local programme, or could be referred to another transplant centre for this type of operation.

The procedure with this type of transplant involves being attached to a machine, rather like haemodialysis, to remove antibodies before having the transplant, so there is no risk of the body attacking or rejecting the kidney soon after the operation. This treatment is called plasmapheresis and usually lasts 10 days. If you need it, you will be treated by machine every other day in addition to your usual dialysis regimen. After the transplant, stronger immunosuppressant drugs than usual may be used, as well as more sessions on the machine.

There is still a risk of rejection, mostly in the first two weeks after the transplant operation. If this occurs, much stronger treatment is required to treat the rejection than in 'standard' transplants. Even if this is successful, there is a higher risk of complications.

After the first three months, the transplant seems to behave like a 'standard' kidney transplant, and treatment is given as normal. In some cases antibodies return, but the kidney seems to adapt and not be harmed by them.

The risk of death or transplant failure if you and your donor are 'antibody incompatible' is about twice that of a 'standard' transplant. It is important that you have a chance to talk this through in detail with your doctor, your donor, and a counsellor.

'EXCHANGE' OR 'PAIRED DONOR' TRANSPLANTATION

The most recent development to try to get around antibody incompatibility (whether for antibodies or blood group compatibility) is paired donation, or exchange transplantation. For example, if a patient is blood group A and has a potential living donor who is blood group B, then there is a blood group barrier to transplantation – and a transplant will not normally be possible. If there is another patient who is blood group B, and

---

SURESH: ANTIBODY IMCOMPATIBLE TRANSPLANT

Suresh has been a kidney patient for 15 years. He has had two kidney transplants during this time, and has been on dialysis for a total of six years in-between. Both transplants came from deceased donors. Unfortunately the second transplant failed quite soon after the operation due to a blood clot and Suresh has had to go back onto haemodialysis three times a week in hospital. The dialysis does not suit him well. It leaves him quite tired and, as he lives a distance from the hospital, he has had to leave his job as a computer programmer. He is desperate for another transplant.

Suresh's wife Meena agrees to donate a kidney and, following tests, is found to be a suitable donor. Unfortunately Suresh has very high antibody levels directed against the tissue type of his wife, which might cause severe rejection after a transplant. In order for him to be able to have the kidney from his wife he must first have plasmapheresis every other day over the 10 days before the transplant in addition to his haemodialysis treatment. Although this treatment is disruptive, exhausting and painful, Suresh and Meena both feel that it will be worth it in the long term - if it means that her kidney donation will be successful.

The transplant operation is straightforward and the new kidney works well for the first week. Then Suresh's levels of antibodies rise and there is a rejection episode, with the transplant passing less urine and his blood creatinine level rising. After five days of intensive anti-rejection treatment, the kidney recovers. Three months after the transplant, Suresh feels well, and is on much lower doses of anti-rejection drugs. Indeed, he is on much the same doses as anyone else who has an uncomplicated transplant.

---

who has a living donor who is blood group A, they will also be incompatible. However, if each donor allowed their kidneys to be transplanted into the other patient, then two uncomplicated, blood group compatible, transplants could take place. To perform two 'normal' transplants is much simpler and safer from a medical point of view than doing two antibody incompatible transplants. It is also likely to give both patients a better chance of a transplant that works well for longer.

There are two drawbacks to paired donor transplantation. First, not many donor and patient pairs are blood group A and B. The common blood group in the UK is type O, and someone who is blood group O can donate to someone of any blood group. Second, half the people who have antibody incompatibility with their donors have antibodies against tissue types, not blood groups (some of course have both).

To find another donor and patient for an exchange may not be easy if the patient has tissue type antibodies, because many patients have antibodies against lots of people. In other words, they could reject kidneys from many other people, as well as from the friend or relative who has offered to donate to them personally. Finding a match may be very difficult.

In order to get round this problem, exchange transplants are organised on a national basis in the UK. People willing to go through with an exchange are registered onto a central database, and a computer-matching run is performed on a regular basis to see who matches up.

An important consideration in exchange transplantation is to maintain anonymity between the two sets of donor and patient. So if you are hoping to go through with an exchange transplant, you will not know anything about the other pair. Also, the two transplant operations will take place simultaneously (generally in different hospitals, which may or may not be close to each other).

ALTERNATIVES TO ANTIBODY INCOMPATIBLE AND EXCHANGE TRANSPLANTATION

Alternatives to AIT and exchange transplantation include waiting for a deceased donor kidney, which may be a long wait especially if you have lots of antibodies. If you have tissue type antibodies rather than a blood group problem, a compatible deceased donor kidney could come along.

Occasionally, someone else in the family comes forward to be considered as a living donor, and they turn out to be antibody compatible. In such a case, a 'standard' transplant can be performed.

It is also worth remembering that the results of AIT are improving rapidly. Some people opt to wait for a while and see whether their chances of a successful AIT improve.

GIVING A KIDNEY TO SOMEONE YOU HAVE NEVER MET

So far, we have talked about living donor transplantation in the situation where the donor and recipient have a close relationship with each other. However there are some circumstances, other than paired exchange, where a donor may give a kidney to someone they have never met.

Some people feel strongly that they want to help someone with kidney failure, irrespective of who they are, and will just donate a kidney without knowing who the recipient of the transplant will be. This is called non-

---

EXCHANGE TRANSPLANTATION OR ANTIBODY INCOMPATIBLE TRANSPLANTATION?

Antibody incompatible transplantation has 'taken off' as a specialised but fairly routine procedure as an alternative to exchange transplantation; but there are markedly different views about which is the best way to proceed.

Some people say that AIT is risky, with increased risk of death and transplant failure early after the transplant, and that the long-term results are uncertain. In other words, will any of these transplants work for over 10 years? The early post-transplant period for exchange transplants is so straightforward in the majority of cases that every effort should be made to develop this type of transplantation, rather than AIT.

On the other hand, supporters of AIT point out that many people who go forward for an exchange transplant will not get one, because a match cannot be found. The experience in Holland, and computer modelling in the US, suggest that 50% of people who go forwards for an exchange transplant will not get one, and an AIT is their only realistic chance of getting a living donor transplant.

Some people are cautious about giving a transplant to someone they have never met; and, as the results of AIT improve, they may wish to stick with their own donor-patient combination.

One factor to consider here is the chance of getting a match for an exchange transplant. If the donor is blood group A and the recipient is blood group B, it is probably better to go for an exchange transplant, since you would normally expect to match up with another blood group B and A combination. And, if you have high antibody levels against your donor, AIT may be very risky. But if you have to wait a long time for an exchange transplant, it would be better to go ahead with a high risk AIT.

So the decision about which type of transplant to have depends very much on individual circumstances. You should be given every opportunity for careful discussion and support to help you make the best decision for you.

---

directed 'altruistic' donation. It has only become possible in the UK because of changes in the regulations under the Human Tissue Act (2006), but in other parts of the world this type of transplant has been performed for some years. There are not many altruistic donors, and they are usually motivated by factors such as having a relative who lived a normal life with only one kidney, or knowing someone who had a serious illness and never received a transplant. Research into how donors feel after the operation indicates a very high level of satisfaction, people feeling that the donation has made them a better person. Altruistic donors require very careful assessment including a mandatory mental health assessment and independent assessment before the HTA can give approval for a transplant to proceed.

Another circumstance in which someone can give a kidney to someone they have never met is when kidneys are swapped or exchanged between pairs of donor and recipients to avoid antibody barriers to transplantation. This was discussed in more detail on pages 60–62.

BUYING AND SELLING ORGANS

In the UK, it is illegal to buy or sell kidneys for transplant. There must be no pressure (financial or otherwise) put on to any potential donor to donate, or recipient to accept.

There are many issues to consider when thinking about donating or accepting a living donor transplant. On balance, the results are very good for both the donor and the recipient in well over 90% of people. Many renal units in the UK now encourage patients to think about having a living donor transplant if a suitable donor can be found.

WHAT'S WRONG WITH BUYING A KIDNEY ABROAD?

As it is so hard for someone to get a deceased donor kidney in the UK, why is it wrong to buy a kidney abroad?

This is a very complex matter, upon which there are many different views. Most people, and most doctors, find it morally unacceptable to buy or sell any organ. They feel it devalues human life, which is precious, and may lead to even more unacceptable behaviour (e.g. using children in orphanages as 'organ farms'). They feel there ought to be better ways of helping poor people financially.

But, as other parts of human beings can be bought or sold, e.g. eggs, sperm and blood, why are solid organs any different? Indeed, we would not question someone's right to use their body in other ways for making money, for example fashion modelling or sport (e.g. boxing) that we know may lead to harm. This would be infringing on their human rights. There is a view that human life is precious, and that living donation is fairly safe, so that encouraging transplantation by any means is a good thing.

Ethical concerns include worries about middlemen exploiting poorer people. There have also been suggestions of government-controlled schemes, with governments setting the price and controlling the process.

The main reason why most doctors do not approve of buying organs is that the results are not usually good. Several studies show that patients who bought kidneys overseas, usually in India or Pakistan, had very poor results. Nearly half the patients died or their transplants failed, and many of those who survived with a functioning transplant had serious problems such as hepatitis, HIV and other viral or fungal infections.

YUSUF: DOES IT MAKE SENSE TO BUY ABROAD?

Yusuf lives in Woking where he has a good job in local government and is well-respected by the local community. By the time he reached 50, he had been on haemodialysis for seven years. Even though he had had very high blood pressure (the cause of his kidney failure), he prided himself with keeping fit. After a very careful transplant work-up, including a cardiac catheter (which was normal) he had been put on the transplant waiting list six years ago. He bided his time, took his tablets carefully and followed the tight fluid restriction (less than one litre a day); and never bothered the doctors. After five years on the waiting list, one day he asked his consultant why he had never had an offer of a kidney. He had read on the Internet that the average waiting time for a kidney was 'about 2 years'. The consultant said that it was (a), bad luck and (b), because he was Asian and therefore had a rare tissue type which meant it was difficult to find a suitable match.

At this point Yusuf's wife Zainab asked whether she might be able to give him one of her kidneys, but unfortunately investigations revealed she had previously undiagnosed Type 2 diabetes which made this impossible. Apart from his children, from whom he feels it would be morally wrong to take a kidney, Yusuf has no other relatives living in the UK except his mother, a frail lady in her early 70s.

After another year of waiting, Yusuf had had enough. Against his wife's wishes, he went to Pakistan and bought a kidney. Although deeply unhappy about his decision, Zainab insisted on accompanying him and it turned out to be just as well she did. After ten days, Yusuf developed a severe infection that caused the kidney to fail. He became very ill and believes it was only Zainab's determination to get him the best possible care that saved his life. So he returned home, weakened and shaken, to go back onto dialysis.

To make matters worse, some routine blood tests when he came home revealed that Yusuf had been infected with hepatitis C, presumably from the donor. It is unlikely he will ever be able to have another transplant now. He has to be isolated in a side room for his haemodialysis sessions. He feels like a leper.

Yusuf often thinks about the donor. Was he all right? Did he know he was probably carrying this virus? Has the money he received helped him look after his family? Yusuf doesn't even know whether the donor is still alive, though he thinks it unlikely.

Yusuf feels angry and let down: let down by what he sees as an unfair and racist system of kidney allocation in the UK, and by the purchase of a kidney which has turned out to do more harm than good. Zainab has become depressed and withdrawn. Her husband feels she blames him for buying the kidney in the first place. He misses the warmth there used to be between them.

KEY FACTS

❶ Having a kidney transplant from a living donor is becoming more common and the outlook is good for both the donor and the recipient.

❷ Living donor transplantation is not necessarily straightforward. The emotional and ethical issues around it can be complicated and difficult to deal with.

❸ Donors will have to have be assessed by the Human Tissue Authority to ensure that they are donating their organ freely.

❹ If you have tissue type antibodies (or the 'wrong' blood group) that would make a transplant difficult, you may be helped by a recently developed technique called antibody incompatible transplantation (AIT). This can help your body to accept a kidney from a living donor who is a less than perfect match.

⑤ Another way round problems with matching is for your transplant coordinator to arrange for a 'paired exchange' with another donor-recipient pair.

⑥ Doctors would not encourage buying kidneys from abroad, or going abroad to have a transplant, because of ethical worries and also because the recipient can end up with serious medical problems.

7
The transplant operation

This chapter describes what happens during a kidney transplant operation, and what to expect in hospital afterwards.

Transplanting a kidney is a straightforward operation, with a good success rate. The principles have not changed much since the 1950s, when the first kidney transplants were being pioneered in America. Once you have had a transplant, you will need to take medication every day for the rest of your life. If your transplant fails, you can go back to dialysis or possibly have another transplant. This applies whether your original transplant has come from either a deceased or a living donor.

BRIAN: WHAT IF THE OPERATION CAN'T GO AHEAD?

Brian is 53 years old and has diabetes. He had always been a little overweight though in his early thirties he gained more weight than he ought. Life was great; he was happily married with two children and he was earning good money as a salesman. His eating habits weren't under control though, eating whenever and wherever he could. His weight had ballooned up to 18 stone but he wasn't too worried as his work and family life were fine. At the age of 42 he developed Type 2 diabetes, initially treated by tablets. However 6 months after starting treatment he had to learn how to inject himself twice a day with insulin. When he was 50 he developed kidney failure as a result of his diabetes and he started peritoneal dialysis. Unfortunately, after a year, he had a few problems with his dialysis and he had to transfer to haemodialysis treatments three times a week at the renal unit about 10 miles from his home.

Brian's wife Carol wanted to give him a kidney but she was also overweight and therefore not a suitable donor. His children were too young to become donors. However, as Brian now weighed 18 stone, he was told he was not suitable for any form of transplant, either deceased or living donor.

The thought of a transplant gave Brian the motivation to get fitter and lose some weight. It took him two years to get down to 14 stone. He had all the relevant tests and was placed on deceased donor list.

He had only been on the transplant list for a year when he 'got the call' and was told there was a kidney available for him. He tried not to panic but made his way swiftly to the hospital. Almost as soon as he arrived, his blood was sent to the lab to check the cross-match with the donated kidney. He was excited but anxious. After a careful examination by a junior doctor, then an anaesthetist, he was told he was fit enough for the operation. The surgeon, dressed in theatre greens, popped in to say 'hello' and told him it was a 'very good kidney'. An hour later, he was ready to go to theatre. It was then that a nurse came into his room to give him some bad news. Unfortunately the cross-match was positive and it was predicted that he would probably reject the kidney almost as soon as it was transplanted. Brian was devastated. He had a cup of sweet tea, got dressed, and Carol drove him home. They stopped in a lay-by near the front of the hospital and cried. They noticed a car driving into the hospital with two people in it. Was one of them another patient who would get the kidney? Brian hoped so, and wished them luck.

THE OPERATION

An operation to transplant a kidney lasts about 2–3 hours and you will need a general anaesthetic. You may be away from the ward for 5–6 hours in total. This is because of the time you will need to spend in the anaesthetic room before the operation and in the recovery room afterwards. To start the operation the surgeon will make a diagonal incision (cut) into your abdomen, on the right or the left, below the navel (see Figure 7.1). The incision may be straight or curved, depending on the usual practice in your hospital. The curved incisions are sometimes called 'hockey stick' incisions because of their shape.

The surgeon will leave your existing kidneys where they are. They won't cause any harm and removing them is unnecessary. The transplant kidney will be placed lower down in your abdomen, just above the groin (see Figure 7.3). The transplant kidney has its own artery (to take blood to it), vein (to take blood from it) and ureter (to take urine to your bladder).

The artery belonging to the new kidney will be attached to your main artery supplying blood to the leg on that side of your body. The vein belonging to the new kidney will be attached to the main vein carrying blood from that leg. These leg blood vessels are big enough to be able to send blood to and from the new kidney without affecting the blood supply to the leg. The transplant kidney's ureter will be attached to your own

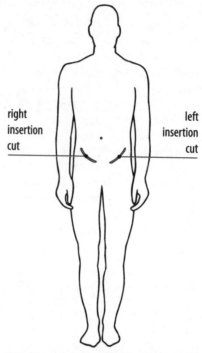

right   left
insertion   insertion
cut   cut

Figure 7.1 Incision sites for transplant operation (note: only one cut will be made, on either the right or the left side of the abdomen, depending on which side the kidney will be inserted)

bladder. A small plastic pipe (called a double J stent) is usually inserted into the ureter (see Figure 7.2) to help prevent the ureter from becoming blocked after the operation. At the end of the operation, your abdomen will be closed with stitches.

AFTER THE OPERATION

When you wake up from the anaesthetic after the transplant operation, you will find you have several tubes coming out of your body. These will include:

- A urinary catheter (a tube into your bladder);

- A central venous pressure tube (CVP) (which is placed in the side of your neck, and measures the pressure of blood inside your heart);

- An intravenous drip in your arm (to give you fluid and drugs if necessary);

- One or more thin plastic tubes (surgical drains) coming out of your abdomen, to drain off any fluid that gathers around your kidney after the operation.

These tubes will be removed one by one over the next few days. The urinary catheter is usually left in place for around 5 days. The double J stent is usually removed during a small operation (under local or general anaesthetic) about three months after the transplant. If you have been on peritoneal dialysis, your PD catheter will probably be removed at the same time. If you have been on haemodialysis, your fistula may stop working at some stage after the transplant. This does not matter, provided your transplant is working well.

The first few days after the operation are crucial, and you will be monitored very closely. Your blood pressure will be monitored with great care, and a close watch will be kept on how much liquid you drink and how

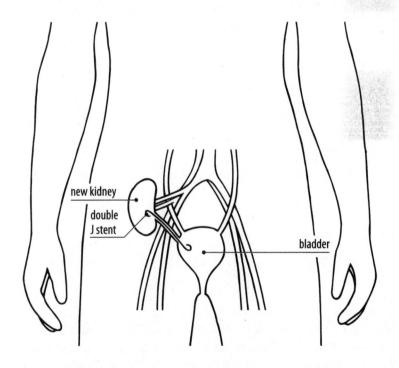

new kidney

double
J stent

bladder

Figure 7.2 Double J stent, shown in position

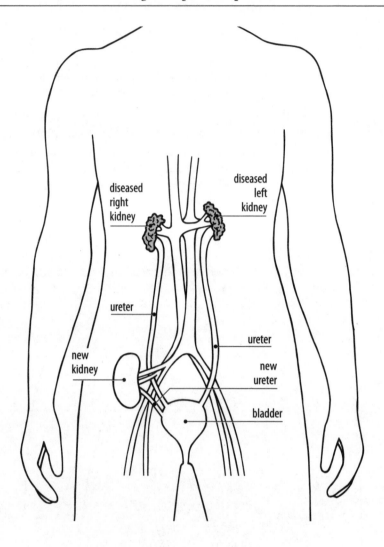

Figure 7.3 New kidney in position (right insertion)

much urine you pass. Many patients will be able to drink and eat small amounts, and sit out of bed, the day after the operation.

Pain relief is very important, and you should know how you will be able to get this. You can be given injections or tablets. In many hospitals, patients can control their own pain relief by giving themselves frequent small doses of a strong painkiller. This is done using a special injection pump (called a PCA pump, see page 50) which is controlled by pressing a button on a wristband. Before your operation, ask whether this form of pain relief will be available at your transplant unit, and make sure someone shows you how to operate the machine before you have the operation.

Expect to have blood tests to measure your blood creatinine level measured every day while you are in hospital following your transplant. The lower your creatinine level is, the better. This tells the doctors how well or not your transplant kidney is working. The amount of urine that the new kidney makes will not be a reliable indicator, as people who have just had a transplant may produce a large volume of urine that does not contain many wastes.

In about one third of kidney transplant patients (more if the kidney has come from a non-heartbeating donor – see page 23), the kidney does not produce any urine for the first few days (and sometimes for the first few weeks) after the transplant operation. This does not mean that the transplant will never work – sometimes they take time to 'get going' and are referred to as 'sleeping kidneys'. This can be very stressful for patients, but

---

MARGARET: A NEW WOMAN

Margaret is 58 and a retired teacher. She 'got the call' one Saturday morning – the last thing she expected as she had only been on the transplant list for 11 months. Her first response on hearing the phone ring was to ignore it, as she was just about to go out shopping. But fortunately she picked up the receiver and her mood changed to a mixture of panic and excitement as she was given the news. 'I didn't know what to do first' she told her daughter Charlotte later. 'Jump straight into the car or phone your Dad!'

The operation went well, and Margaret woke up back on the ward in what seemed no time at all. Over the next few days, she felt as if a fog was lifting. 'It's funny,' she says, 'when you are on dialysis I think you get used to feeling slightly below par, all the time. It's not until you have a transplant that you realise how fuzzy you've been feeling.'

Margaret and her family were amazed at the speed of her recovery. After a good night's sleep, she was out of bed and within two days most of the drips had been removed. Now, six months later, she still can't believe how much better she feels than she did while on dialysis. Neither can her family. Her husband Dave says, 'She's like a new woman. Or rather, it is as if I've got the girl I married back again.'

your doctor should take the time to explain to you that most sleeping kidneys 'wake up' after a few days or a couple of weeks. If your transplant doesn't work at the beginning, you will need to continue on dialysis and play a waiting game until it does start working. A 'good transplant' is one that is working well after one year or more, not two weeks.

HEADING HOME

You should expect to stay in hospital for up to two weeks after the operation. Once you have left hospital, you will need to make a lot of clinic visits over many months. To start with, your doctor will expect to see you at the outpatient clinic three times a week, then twice a week, then once a week, then once every two weeks, and so on. Eventually, when your doctors are satisfied that your transplanted kidney is working well, the time between your appointments may be extended to three months or so. This is usually at the start of the kidney's third year inside you, but may vary depending upon follow-up arrangements in your particular centre.

You will take time to get your energy levels back after a transplant operation, so expect it to be 3–6 months before your feel ready to return to normal activities, including work. However, after either a living donor or a deceased donor transplant, you will probably be encouraged to take gentle exercise (e.g. walking) as soon as possible after the operation. This will help your recovery and also boost your morale as long as you don't overdo it. Transplant patients are recommended not to drive for at least one month after the operation. Neither the function of your new kidney, nor your risk of infection, will be affected by having sex. Even so, it is probably best not to resume sexual activity until about four weeks after leaving hospital. If you are a woman, your fertility may return very quickly. So, if you are of child-bearing age, you should start using contraception as soon as you resume sexual activity. Women are normally advised to avoid getting pregnant in the first year after a transplant.

KEY FACTS

1. Transplanting a kidney is a straightforward operation, with a good success rate.

2. The new kidney is placed in the patient's groin area. This is a convenient place to connect it to a blood supply and the bladder.

3. The patient's own kidneys are usually left in place.

4. The operation usually takes 2–3 hours.

5. The first few days after the operation are very important. Your health and kidney function will be monitored closely.

6. Sometimes the kidney doesn't work right way. This does not mean that it will never work. You may need to have dialysis until it 'wakes up'.

7. Most patients can go home about two weeks after the operation.

8
Medication

This chapter tells you about the tablets you will be given after your transplant operation, especially the various immunosuppressant drugs. The reason why you need all this medication is explained, as is the importance of taking it regularly.

All patients who have a kidney transplant need to take drugs called immunosuppressant drugs. As the name 'immunosuppressant' suggests, the function of these drugs is to suppress your immune system. The aim is to dampen down the immune system just enough to stop it rejecting the transplant kidney, while still keeping it active enough to fight infection. Finding the right balance can be difficult.

HOW IMMUNOSUPPRESSANT DRUGS WORK

Several different drugs are used to prevent rejection in a kidney transplant. Transplant doctors prescribe these drugs to patients in a variety of ways, depending on their personal preferences. This does not matter; the results of different drug protocols are similar.

All immunosuppressant drugs work by changing the way white blood cells behave in the body. White blood cells help to fight infection and foreign bodies (such as splinters and, of course, transplants). By altering the way that white blood cells work, the body will be less able to fight infection and foreign bodies. This might mean that you will catch a cold more easily, but it also means that your body is less likely to reject the transplanted kidney.

The drugs affect white blood cells in different ways. Some drugs are very similar to others, so there is no point in using two drugs from the same 'group' at the same time. Using more than one immunosuppressive drug from different groups at the same time can have a more powerful immunosuppressant effect. This can also help reduce the side effects, because each drug can be used in a lower dose than if it was used on its own. Having several different types of drug available also means that people can change between different drugs if they don't work well enough for them. It is also useful for people to be able to change drugs if they experience side effects. It is easiest to explain the ways the different drugs work by using an example. Let us imagine that the white blood cell is a motor car . . .

Group 1 – 'The Brakes'
(ciclosporin and tacrolimus)
These stop white blood cells 'activating' and rejecting, a bit like putting the brake on in a car so it cannot move. Most people with kidney transplants receive either ciclosporin or tacrolimus (but not both together). Sirolimus is another drug that stops white blood cells activating, but works slightly differently from ciclosporin and tacrolimus, and has a different side effects (see page 79).

Group 2 – 'The Secret Policemen'
(azathioprine and mycophenolate mofetil)
These drugs kill cells that are trying to cause rejection. This is rather like an over-enthusiastic policeman stopping your car for speeding and taking it away to be crushed. Again, most people receive one or the other of these drugs, not both.

Group 3 – 'The Bad Mechanic'
(prednisolone, a steroid drug)
This reduces the activity of a lot of cells in the body, having an overall 'damping down' effect, like a bad mechanic de-tuning the car's engine. There is no alternative drug to prednisolone.

Group 4 – 'The Keys'
(basiliximab or daclizumab)
These drugs block activating signals reaching white blood cells, rather like the car doors being locked with the keys inside when you want to go somewhere. One of these drugs may be given by injection at the time of a transplant and again a few days later.

Most patients will start treatment with a Group 1 drug and probably stay on that drug along with a Group 2 drug, forever. Most patients will also be prescribed prednisolone; however many patients are asked to stop taking this after a year if the transplant is working well.

TYPES OF IMMUNOSUPPRESSANT DRUGS AND THEIR SIDE EFFECTS

Group 1: ciclosporin and tacrolimus

These are the most important drugs used to prevent kidney rejection, and work in a similar way to each other. They are given in tablet form, and must be taken every day. One or other of these two drugs (but not both together) will be given to nearly everyone having a kidney transplant in the UK. Unfortunately, if patients are given too much of either ciclosporin or tacrolimus, it can prevent the transplant from working. This is because both drugs can be toxic (poisonous) to the kidney if they are not used with great care. This condition is called ciclosporin (or tacrolimus) toxicity.

To reduce the risk of problems, patients on either of these drugs will have the amount of the drug in their blood monitored by regular blood tests. The blood level that doctors use to check that the right dose is being prescribed is the level just before the next dose is taken. So, if you are having bloods taken to monitor your transplant, do not take your ciclosporin or tacrolimus until after the blood test has been done. If you forget and take the tablets, the blood level of the drug will be higher than expected. Tell the transplant clinic if you have done this, so they can take account of the high level and won't change your drug doses on the basis of misleading results.

The desired blood level of the drug is different at different times after a transplant. For example in the first six months, preventing rejection is paramount. So higher levels are tolerated when compared to after a year, for example. At this time, reducing the toxicity of the drug may be more important, and different units use different target levels. This is why we have not given you 'desired levels' in this book.

Some patients who take ciclosporin for a long time develop a condition called gum hypertrophy (swelling of the gums). This is an excessive growth of the gums, which can be unsightly. If the problem becomes severe, your gums can be 'cut back' using a specialist hospital-based dental treatment. It is less likely to develop if you practise good dental hygiene, including regular brushing and flossing between your teeth.

Another possible side effect of ciclosporin is excessive growth of hair on your face and body. This can be more of a problem for women than men. Tacrolimus does not cause gum swelling or increased hair growth, but it can cause hair loss and trembling. Both drugs can cause diabetes, but tacrolimus does so more often (in up to 15% of patients).

Ciclosporin and tacrolimus can both affect nerves in the body. The most common symptom is shaking of the hands (a tremor). This is most marked when the blood levels of the drug are too high. The tremor is likely to get better, or least improve, when the dose of the drug is reduced. Changes in the doses of the drug should be as recommended by your transplant clinic.

DO NOT change your drug doses by yourself!

A few patients get pins and needles or numbness in their hands and feet. This could be because of ciclosporin or tacrolimus, but could also be because of something else such as diabetes. If you do get these symptoms, you will need tests to find out the exact cause.

A number of patients say that they get a lot of headaches after a transplant, or have muddled thinking. In some cases this may be due to the drugs, but the same symptoms can also be caused by stress or depression, so changing the doses of immunosuppressant drugs will not necessarily help.

Sirolimus
This drug is not so poisonous to the kidney. However, it does have side effects, especially problems with healing, and a very high cholesterol (a type of fat) level in the blood. Therefore it is often not started until some time after the transplant, at the same time that other drugs are reduced in dose (or stopped). Another tablet, called a statin, will be given if your cholesterol level rises.

Group 2: azathioprine and mycophenolate mofetil
Nearly everyone who has a kidney transplant in the UK will be given either azathioprine or mycophenolate, but not both at the same time. These drugs slow down the rate at which new blood cells can be made, and this can cause a number of serious problems. If too few red blood cells are produced, you will suffer from anaemia and become very tired. If you have too few white blood cells, you will develop a condition called neutropenia (a shortage of white blood cells). Neutropenia affects the body's ability to fight infection. If too few of the blood cells called platelets are produced, the resulting problem is thrombocytopenia, which can cause an increased tendency to bleed.

If you are taking either of these drugs, you may suffer from any or all of the above problems. Stopping the drug or reducing the dose will normally put matters right. However, this should only be done under guidance from your doctor. If you stop the pills on your own, without the right advice or monitoring, this may cause your kidney to fail because of rejection.

DO NOT change your drug doses by yourself!

Azathioprine can also cause damage to the liver, so if you are taking it you will have regular blood tests to watch out for any damage. Mycophenolate mofetil can cause gastrointestinal problems, particularly abdominal pain and diarrhoea.

Group 3: prednisolone

This drug is a steroid. Like other steroid drugs, it can cause thinning of the skin which leads to easy bruising, acne and facial swelling (giving a red and rounded appearance to the face). Steroids can also cause you to gain weight, and they weaken your bones, making you more likely to fracture your vertebrae (the bones of the spine) or hips.

There is more about bone health in Chapter 10.

Like ciclosporin and tacrolimus, prednisolone can also cause diabetes mellitus ('sugar diabetes'). At worst, this might mean that that you would have to take tablets or give yourself insulin injections twice a day. Diabetes can also damage kidneys if it is not well controlled.

Another possible problem with prednisolone is that it can cause bone damage in the joints, especially the hip joints. Pain in either hip, even in the first 3–6 months after a transplant, should be taken seriously. Replacement of one or both hips may become necessary if there is a serious problem. In the longer term, patients taking prednisolone are also at increased risk of thinning of the bones (osteoporosis). Because of this, the vertebrae (bones of the spine) can collapse causing a 'crush fracture'. This can be very painful, as well as reducing your height. If you are taking prednisolone, you should have your bone density measured at least once a year, using a DEXA scan (see Chapter 10). If there is any sign of bone thinning, then a tablet can be prescribed to strengthen the bones.

Some doctors try to withdraw steroid tablets after the first 12 months because of these side effects on the joints and bones. This usually causes the creatinine to rise by 10 μmol/L (micromoles per litre of blood) or so, which is not usually a problem. But it does carry a very small risk of rejection (or even loss) of the kidney. Stopping the steroids could cause some scarring or fibrosis in the new kidney. This is why many transplant units will leave people on a small dose of steroids, and only withdraw fully if there are clear side effects from them, that is to say if the small risk of complete withdrawal is balanced by a definite benefit in that particular person.

When steroids are withdrawn or the dose is reduced, some people get a steroid withdrawal syndrome. This is because natural steroids are essential to health, and taking tablets of steroid can reduce the body's ability to produce its own natural steroids. Steroid withdrawal syndrome consists of feeling run down, with aches and pains in joints and muscles, and sometimes depression. Usually it resolves if you 'tough it out' for a couple of weeks, but sometimes the steroid dose has to be put back up. Some people have to stay on steroid tablets for life.

SHOULD STEROIDS (PREDNISOLONE) BE USED AFTER TRANSPLANTATION?

There is much debate about whether patients should be prescribed steroids at all after a transplant operation. They are strong drugs with a lot of unpleasant side effects. It is true that they can help to prevent the body rejecting the kidney transplant, but it is unclear whether they affect the long-term survival of the new kidney. This is partly because they are now used in combination with newer and better drugs. Nonetheless, most UK units use them for the first year after the transplant and then consider stopping them slowly if the transplant is working well. A few units do not use steroids in every patient, but might prescribe them (to about 30% of patients) if they get more than one episode of rejection.

Steroid-free transplantation is being offered routinely in some parts of the UK, and most units would try steroid-free treatment if a patient asked for it. The problem is that steroids really do make a difference in lowering the number of rejection episodes. For this reason, the standard advice from the American Society of Transplantation is still to use steroid treatment. This advice is based on a number of research studies where people have been allocated to different treatment regimes after transplantation.

Group 4: basiliximab and daclizumab

You will be given one of these drugs by injection just before and just after your transplant operation. They are not given by tablet and you do not really need to remember the name of the drug! They work in a similar way, so you will be given one or the other but not both. These drugs halve the risk of your body rejecting the kidney early on, while having very few side effects.

Another drug given by injection around the time of the transplant, called alemtuzumab (or Campath), is currently in research trials and may be used routinely in some patients in the near future. Alemtuzumab kills cells rather than inactivating them, so it is probably 'stronger'. It is early days yet, but this might allow other drugs to be used in lower doses. It might also be effective in protecting complicated transplants such as kidney-pancreas grafts.

WORKING OUT WHAT IS BEST FOR YOU

Although transplant units have a standard combination of drugs that they will prescribe to most patients at the time of the transplant, there will be a number of changes to this combination. Even if all the individual drugs stay the same, their doses will be reduced gradually over a period of time to a 'maintenance' dose. If you have a rejection episode on a combination of drugs, you may be given a 'stronger' drug to reduce the chances of further rejection episodes. For example, if someone taking tacrolimus, azathioprine and prednisolone had a rejection episode, the azathioprine might be changed to mycophenolate which is 'stronger'.

WHICH COMBINATION OF IMMUNOSUPPRESSANT DRUGS IS THE MOST EFFECTIVE?

This is probably the most controversial area in transplant medicine. There is no best combination of immunosuppressant drugs but a wide range is now available. The National Institute for Health and Clinical Excellence (NICE, see Appendix 1) has produced guidelines that advise transplant doctors on the most effective use of immunosuppressant drugs following a kidney transplant. The advice from NICE is to give patients a one-off injection of either basiliximab or daclizumab to suppress their immune system immediately after transplant surgery. This drug is not given again. Patients also receive another drug such as ciclosporin (a drug that has been around since the 1980s) or tacrolimus (also called FK506). Ciclosporin and tacrolimus are similar drugs, but tacrolimus is slightly more powerful and works better to prevent the kidney transplant being rejected. However, as it is a stronger medicine, patients tend to get more side effects, especially diabetes, which can be permanent. Some doctors prefer to prescribe ciclosporin, as it has fewer side effects, whereas others prefer tacrolimus as it is more effective.

Drug regimes should be tailored to the patient's specific needs and treatment requirements. The patient should be kept fully informed about which drugs are to be given and what side effects might be expected. Patients should also be allowed to make choices where appropriate. Most units would gently resist a change to the standard drugs they use early on, but would be more flexible after the first 3 months.

The other reason for changing drugs might be side effects. If, for example, you are taking ciclosporin and developed very swollen gums that did not respond to a reduction in the ciclosporin dose, then your prescription might be changed to tacrolimus which also stops the transplant from rejecting but which does not have this side effect. Also, if you are taking prednisolone tablets and you are getting problems, it might be possible to stop the steroids. There is not an alternative drug to switch to, but the dose of one of the other anti-rejection drugs might be kept at a slightly higher level to compensate for stopping the steroids.

SUKI: GETTING THE COMBINATION RIGHT

Suki was a beautiful Asian girl who developed kidney failure for no apparent reason. The doctors said her kidneys were small and may have been defective since she was born. Suki preferred to have haemodialysis, as she was afraid PD would make her stomach stick out. She hid the fistula on her left wrist under some bangles and hoped no one would know she was 'a kidney patient'.

Delicately built and proud of her slim figure, Suki weighed just 7 stone. She wore a belly button stud on her flat tummy and had already started a career in modelling.

After six months on dialysis, Suki was offered a kidney and this worked well from the start. Unfortunately, the steroid tablets made her put on nearly 3 stone in weight – a huge proportion of her existing body weight. The ciclosporin made her gums swell and gave her bad breath. It also caused her to develop facial hair, to the extent that she now has to shave

(Asian people are often prone to this particular side effect). Suki felt that no one had taken the trouble to talk through potential side effects with her before the operation. Some of the doctors in the clinic suggested she changed to drugs that were less likely to give her these side effects. Others were less helpful and seemed to think she was being ungrateful, and should just feel lucky to have received a transplant when so many other people were waiting. She lost confidence in the medical profession and was frightened to change to another tablet regime in case it made things worse or caused her to lose the kidney.

The transplant nurse picked up Suki's concerns. She was able to reassure Suki by telling her that many other patients did change their immuno-suppressant drugs because of side effects, and that this could be very successful. She arranged for Suki to talk to another woman who had experienced cosmetic problems after a transplant, and who had improved after changing the drugs. Suki decided to try and change the drugs, and the doctors in clinic gave her a schedule to change from ciclosporin to tacrolimus, and gradually to stop her prednisolone completely. Throughout this changeover, she had very careful monitoring of her blood tests. Now the gum swelling and excess hair growth have disappeared, and Suki has lost most of the weight she put on after the transplant, and her new kidney still has excellent function.

MAKING SURE YOU KNOW WHAT TO EXPECT

Suki was particularly unlucky in the early months, but much of her distress was caused by her feeling that she had been given no advance information about the possible side effects of her drugs. It is very important that your doctors talk through with you the implications of your post-transplant medication. Ideally they should do this when you are first tested for your fitness to go onto the transplant list, and then again when you come in for your cross-match immediately before the transplant operation. You should not only be told about the side effects, but given written information that you can look at and refer to again at home. Nobody remembers everything they are told in the doctor's surgery or clinic.

If you don't feel you are being given the information you need, then ask, and if necessary ask again. You have a right to information about how any treatment you are offered might affect you.

If you have particular concerns – for example, you can't imagine anything worse than gum trouble and bad breath – please do mention this to your doctor at the first opportunity. Ideally, you should have the chance to do this before the drug treatment starts (which is probably before you have the operation). If you feel your doctor is not taking your concerns sufficiently seriously, ask to see another doctor. You have rights, and your agenda must be taken on board as far as possible.

Many people find it helpful to talk to either the transplant nurse or a specialist pharmacist from the transplant centre. They will be able to talk you through all the drug combinations and their possible side effects. They will also be able to tell you about any alternatives.

Once you have been started on a regime of immunosuppressant medication, you should feel free to discuss with your doctor any worries you have about how the drugs are affecting you. Sometimes, side effects settle down. If they persist, the doctor should be able to change one drug for another (ciclosporin to tacrolimus or sirolimus, for example) or look again at the dose levels.

There sometimes seems to be a reluctance to alter medication on an 'if it isn't broke, don't fix it' principle. Some people seem to go for years without any changes in medication levels. If you feel this is the case for you, do speak to your doctor. Government 'Best Practice' recommendations now include a regular review of all the medication you are taking. If you feel you are not being given the correct drug, or if changes to your prescription do not seem to have been continued, or you don't feel your drug regime is being reviewed regularly, you should speak to your doctor or transplant nurse. If you are still worried, you can ring the NKF helpline (see Appendix 2).

CONTINUING YOUR MEDICATION

You should expect to carry on taking tacrolimus or ciclosporin for as long as your transplant continues to function. If neither tacrolimus nor ciclosporin are effective for you, or if you have too many unpleasant side effects, your doctor may prescribe sirolimus for you instead.

You will be given another long-term immunosuppressant drug along with your ciclosporin, tacrolimus or sirolimus. This will probably be azathioprine or mycophenolate mofetil. Azathioprine has been available for many years whereas mycophenolate mofetil is relatively new. Most patients are also prescribed the steroid drug prednisolone in addition to their immunosuppressant drugs (see above).

If you find you are getting side effects from taking these drugs, you should tell your transplant doctor as soon as possible. It may be possible to give you an alternative – for example ciclosporin might be changed for tacrolimus, or azathioprine for mycophenolate mofetil and vice versa.

The choice of drugs is influenced partly by the cost and partly by the long-term side effects. Some doctors are less willing to prescribe newer drugs, as their long-term effects may not yet be fully understood.

In reality, whichever combination of drugs is given, they will be effective at preventing your body's defence mechanisms (immune system) from rejecting your new kidney. What is most important is the attention that your doctors and nurses pay to the effectiveness and possible side effects of the combination of drugs they have chosen for you.

PETER: CREATININE UP – REJECTION OR TACROLIMUS TOXICITY?

Peter, a 39-year-old builder, recovers well from his transplant operation. He is given a one off injection of basiliximab and then prescribed the immunosuppressant drug tacrolimus together with prednisolone and azathioprine which he takes every day. He has no rejection in the first weeks after his transplant and is discharged home after 10 days. Peter has to attend the transplant clinic regularly after the transplant. At each visit the nurse takes blood to check how well the new kidney is working and to make sure that the levels of the drugs in his blood are high enough to prevent rejection, but low enough to minimise side effects.

About six weeks after the operation, he gets a phone call from the transplant nurse who tells him that his blood creatinine level has risen to 180 µmol/L. She tells him that this can be a sign of rejection or it could be caused by the immunosuppressant drug. She gives him specific instructions on a new lower dose and asks him to come back to clinic in two days for more blood tests.

At his next three clinic visits his creatinine level remains high. A decision is made to change Peter's tacrolimus to sirolimus. After a few weeks, his blood creatinine level comes down to 130 µmol/L. It turned out there was no rejection. In fact the reverse was true, in that Peter was receiving so much of an anti-rejection drug that it was toxic to the kidney.

OTHER DRUGS AFTER A TRANSPLANT

Usually, patients who have had a transplant can stop taking some of the drugs that they had before the operation. Most patients can stop having EPO injections and phosphate binding tablets. However, these will be exchanged for two or three of the immunosuppressant drugs described above. You must remember to take your immunosuppressants every day because, if you don't, you will give your immune system the chance to 'fight back' and your body will reject the new kidney. If you are unable to take your immunosuppressant drugs, either because they have run out or because you are suffering from diarrhoea or vomiting, you should go to the hospital at once. The immune system never forgets that there is a 'foreign' kidney in the body. It is always waiting for a chance to attack and reject it.

IMPORTANT

- **If you are unable to take your immunosuppressant medicines for 24 hours or more (either because you feel sick, are vomiting or have diarrhoea, or are ill in some other way, or have run out of tablets), this will have very serious consequences.**

- **Go *straight* to the hospital where your kidney unit team will know how best to manage your situation.**

In addition to your immunosuppressant drugs, you are likely to be given various drugs to prevent infection for about 6–12 months after your operation. You will find more information about this in Chapter 9.

People who have had a kidney transplant need to be very careful about what medicines they take. It is very important always to check that any drugs provided by the hospital, GP, or local pharmacy are *exactly* what is on the prescription. This is particularly important if your kidney doctor has recently changed your treatment.

Many medications, either those that have been prescribed by a doctor or those that have been bought 'over-the-counter' from a chemist, can affect the way that the immunosuppressant drugs work. This is especially important for ciclosporin and tacrolimus, both of which are very 'sensitive' drugs. New medications can cause either of these immuno-suppressants to work too well, which will make them toxic to the kidney transplant. They can also make the immunosuppressant drugs work less well, risking rejection. Either of these interactions can cause the creatinine level to go up. So you should always check with the pharmacist at your kidney unit, or your hospital doctor or transplant nurse before taking anything new or different. It is unfair to ask a GP about drugs that affect immunosuppressants. GPs see hundreds of people all with different health problems so it is unrealistic to expect them to have the specialist knowledge they would need to advise you.

You should *never* assume that just because a medicine or tablet is common and easily available (like aspirin, for example), it is necessarily 'safe' to take if you have had a transplant. You should be equally careful about 'herbal', 'complementary' or 'alternative' medicines or treatments. Some of these, such as St John's Wort, can have considerable effects on the way in which other drugs work, and these can be difficult to predict.

You also need to be aware that grapefruit (or even grapefruit juice) can affect the way your immunosuppressant medication behaves in your body. The safest course is to avoid grapefruit if you can.

KEY FACTS

1. All patients who have a kidney transplant need to take drugs to prevent their body from rejecting the new kidney.

2. These drugs are called immunosuppressant drugs.

3. There are four different groups of drugs that are used in combination.

4. The drugs are powerful and have some unpleasant side effects.

5. Tacrolimus and ciclosporin can be toxic to the kidney; so blood levels must be measured.

6. Azathioprine and mycophenolate suppress the bone marrow where blood cells are made. This results in anaemia (lack of red cells), infections (caused by lack of white cells) and bleeding (caused by lack of platelets).

7. Prednisolone may weaken the bones, which can cause fractures.

8. Transplant doctors can alter the drugs (and the doses) to help reduce the side effects.

9. Transplant patients need to take their drugs every day.

10. If you vomit, have diarrhoea, forget to take a dose or run out of the drugs, you should contact your renal unit immediately.

9
The first three months

This chapter discusses the two most important issues to be aware of in the first few months after a kidney transplant. We explain the process of rejection and talk about infections, both of which might affect your health or the function of your transplant.

Although a kidney transplant is an excellent treatment for most people with ERF, it is not problem-free. In the first three months after a kidney transplant, about 2% of patients will die, and 4% will lose their transplant. Over time, the risk of complications reduces, but they can occur at any time and most transplants will eventually fail. Problems that occur more often after the first three months are discussed in the next chapter.

REJECTION

Some people who have had a transplant experience a problem called 'rejection'. The term rejection is used to describe the process of the body recognising the new transplanted kidney as 'foreign' and using its defences to destroy it.

Many people find even the thought of rejection terrifying, particularly with their first transplant. When it is dealt with efficiently and effectively, you might wonder what all the fuss was about and why you were so worried. Nevertheless, it is important to be aware that your body might reject the new kidney at any time.

THE REJECTION PROCESS

Rejection can occur in any kidney transplant, even when the patient and the transplant kidney are apparently 'well matched' (in terms of blood group and tissue type, see Chapter 2). The severity of rejection varies from patient to patient. Rejection may be either acute or chronic. Acute rejection develops over a period of days, and may cause just a slight rise in the blood creatinine level without any symptoms, or can cause a marked fall in the urine output and a reduction in transplant function. This may mean dialysis is again necessary. This is usually temporary though, as the vast majority of episodes of acute rejection can be treated. Chronic rejection develops slowly over months or years, and is discussed in Chapter 12.

It is the body's immune system that is responsible for the rejection process. The immune system is the body's natural defence system. The immune system isn't in just one part of the body; it is all over the body. Some organs, such as the spleen and the appendix, are part of the immune system. The lymph nodes (or 'glands'), such as those in the neck and under the arms, and specialist white blood cells (called lymphocytes) are also part of the immune system.

The immune system's job is to fight anything that the body does not recognise as its own. This includes germs (such as bacteria and viruses) and foreign objects (such as splinters or thorns embedded in the skin). The body's immune system can also fight cancer. Your immune system does not usually attack parts of your own body because these all have a 'friendly face'. This friendly face is made up of special proteins called antigens, which cover the outer surface of the cells. The immune system recognises the friendly face and knows to leave these cells alone. Germs and foreign objects do not have this friendly face. Cancer cells don't have this friendly face either as they have developed in an abnormal way.

Normally, the immune system is a 'good thing', as it protects the body from dangerous infections, foreign bodies and cancer. However, after a transplant it can be damaging. If the immune system recognises that the new kidney does not have the usual friendly face of the body's own cells, it will become overactive and send lymphocytes (white blood cells) to attack and reject the kidney. The body is actually trying to protect you from the kidney, which it perceives as a danger. Luckily, there are drugs called immunosuppressant drugs (see Chapter 8) that can dampen down the rejection process by suppressing the immune system.

ACUTE REJECTION

'Acute' means short term, coming on quickly and needing immediate action. Acute rejection usually happens in the first three months (particularly the first few weeks) after a transplant. It is very common – about 25% of patients experience acute rejection in the first year after a transplant. If acute rejection hasn't occurred within one year of the operation, then it is unlikely to happen, as long as you take your drugs correctly. However, if you don't take your immunosuppressant drugs, acute rejection can occur at any time. This is why always taking these medicines as prescribed is so important.

Acute rejection may sometimes cause pain and fever and a reduced urine output, but usually there are no symptoms. Doctors will suspect that a patient has acute rejection if the blood creatinine level is either not coming down after a transplant, or if it has started to fall and then remains stable or increases again. However, acute rejection is not the only reason why there may be problems with blood creatinine level after a transplant, and these other possibilities are usually investigated first.

TESTS TO INVESTIGATE REDUCED TRANSPLANT FUNCTION

In the first few months after the transplant operation, your blood creatinine level will be measured regularly. Your creatinine should go down to less than 200 µmol/L. If it goes up, however, this is likely to indicate there is a problem such as your transplanted kidney might be failing. If this happens, your doctors will do a number of tests to investigate the cause of the problem. There are a number of reasons why your creatinine level may increase:

- Acute rejection;

- A problem with the blood supply to your new kidney;

- Dehydration – some kidneys pass too much urine, and it can be hard to drink enough fluid to keep up with the urine output;

- Acute tubular necrosis (the kidney 'going to sleep' shortly after the transplant);

- An infection;

- Problems with the immunosuppressant drugs you are taking (especially if tacrolimus or ciclosporin levels are too high in the blood).

An ultrasound scan might be performed to help find out the cause of the problem. This is a painless test that uses sound waves to look inside the body. It's the same technique that is used to look at the unborn baby when a woman is pregnant. The ultrasound scan will show whether your ureter (the tube that takes urine from the kidney to the bladder) is blocked. You may have another type of scan, for example a nuclear medicine scan or a Doppler scan. Either of these will show if there are any problems with the blood supply to the new kidney.

The only way to be sure whether a transplant kidney is having a rejection episode is to do a transplant kidney biopsy. This involves putting a needle into the transplant kidney and removing a tiny piece. Doctors then look at this under the microscope. If you are having a biopsy, you will need to lie on your back. The biopsy is performed with an ultrasound machine to locate the kidney. It takes only a fraction of a second, but the whole procedure takes about 20 minutes. You will be given an injection of local anaesthetic to numb the skin from where the biopsy is taken, so expect it to be about as painful as having a dental filling. After the biopsy, you will need to lie down for 6–12 hours .

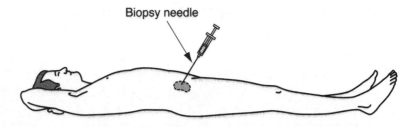

Biopsy needle

Figure 9.1 Having a biopsy of a transplanted kidney

If your biopsy is taken in the morning, the doctor is likely to get the result on the same day. Most patients who have had a kidney transplant will have one or more biopsies in the weeks after the operation.

There are some risks involved with having a kidney biopsy. The main danger after a biopsy is bleeding from the new kidney. There is a 1 in 1000 chance of dying or losing the transplant because of excessive bleeding. However the bleeding is usually not serious and it settles of its own accord.

SHOULD ALL TRANSPLANT RECIPIENTS HAVE ROUTINE BIOPSIES?

Some recent research suggests that everyone who has a kidney transplant should have at least one biopsy in the first month after the transplant, even if the kidney is working perfectly. This is because some biopsies show a low level of a rejection process in the kidney, and treating this may stop any rejection developing, and prevent any long-term damage to the kidney.

Other doctors are more cautious, because of the occasional complications of biopsies, and only perform a biopsy if there is a problem with the kidney function.

In the UK, almost every transplant unit has a slightly different policy for performing biopsies after transplantation. Some perform a biopsy only if there is a problem with the transplant, while some others perform several 'protocol' or routine biopsies at various time points after the transplant. Ask your doctor or transplant nurse what the practice is at your kidney unit.

TREATMENT FOR ACUTE REJECTION

If your biopsy shows signs of kidney rejection, then you are likely to be given a high dose of a steroid drug, either prednisolone or methylprednisolone. The drug is given by tablet or intravenous injection, once a day for three days. These short-course, high-dose treatments are called 'pulses'. This steroid treatment is usually successful as it brings the rejection process under control, and the blood creatinine will start to go down to near normal levels. Occasionally, a patient may need two courses of this (or a similar) drug.

If pulses of prednisolone or methylprednisolone do not work, there are other options. One of the immunosuppressant tablets may be changed to a similar but slightly 'stronger' drug. For example ciclosporin might be stopped and tacrolimus started (see Chapter 8).

Alternatively, you may be given a 5–10 day course of a stronger intravenous injection. The most usual drugs that are used are:

- Anti-thymocyte globulin (ATG);
- Muromonomab-CD3 (OKT3) antibody.

These drugs work in a similar way to the other immunosuppressant drugs but are much more powerful. They work by killing the white blood cells that cause rejection and, as a result, the rejection process goes away. However, they can have fairly severe side effects after the first dose, especially OKT3. These may include fever, diarrhoea, joint and muscle pain, wheezing, and shortness of breath due to fluid on the lungs (pulmonary oedema).

INFECTIONS

People who have just received a transplant are particularly prone to infections, on account of the immunosuppressant drugs that are needed to prevent the body from rejecting the 'new' kidney. These drugs work by

---

MICHAEL: NEVER FORGET
TO TAKE THE IMMUNOSUPPRESSANTS

Michael is a 36-year-old accountant who has a stable kidney transplant for over five years, with a creatinine of about 150 μmol/L. He lives in Durham. One weekend he went to a university friend's wedding near Gloucester. He drove down late on Friday night, after work. He was halfway there (just south of Leeds) when he realised that he had left his tablets at home. As he intended to return Sunday morning, he didn't think it would matter, as he would miss only 4 sets of tablet taking.

The wedding was fun, and he got back about 2pm on the Sunday. To make up for the tablets he missed, he took double doses on the Sunday at 2pm and 10pm.

Michael felt guilty about his decision-making, so he thought he had better have his bloods checked on the following Tuesday. To his astonishment, his creatinine was 280 μmol/L although he felt well. The transplant nurse admitted him that night. He had transplant biopsy on Wednesday, which showed acute rejection. He could not believe it.

Fortunately a three-day course of intravenous methylprednisolone, followed by a week of high dose oral prednisolone, treated the rejection episode. His creatinine slowly returned to his baseline level of 150 μmol/L. Michael now realises that the body never forgets it has a foreign thing inside it, and is always ready to reject it. He will never miss any tablets again.

---

making the immune system less efficient which, in itself, reduces the body's resistance to infections. Although most people will get an infection of some sort after the transplant operation, it is usually not serious.

Because of the publicity surrounding it, the idea of contracting MRSA is particularly frightening for some people. In fact, the chance of catching it is lower than one might think. Many transplant centres have never known cases of MRSA in either donors or recipients. There are some basic precautions you can take however. At the time of your transplant operation, you should let the hospital know if you have ever had MRSA in the past. You should have swabs for MRSA taken as a matter of routine to make sure none is lurking on the skin where it could move over to the wound.

Another bug that makes news headlines, *C. difficile* (which is a diarrhoea bug), can occasionally occur. You can help reduce your chances of getting this by making sure that any course of antibiotics you get is as short as possible – preferably less than 7 days. You can also keep a close eye on hand washing by all hospital workers, including the doctors who come into your room. Unfortunately, people who have other medical conditions such as diabetes, lung disease or polycystic kidneys (which increase the risk of infection) are more likely to develop infections.

Urinary infection
Urine infections affect about half of all people who receive a kidney transplant. Urine infections are more common in people whose kidney failure was originally caused by reflux nephropathy or diabetes. Such infections usually cause pain when passing urine and a feeling of needing to pass urine frequently. More severe urine infections may cause fevers and pain in the transplanted kidney. Urine infections are usually easy to cure with antibiotics, although severe or repeated infections may need a longer course of preventative antibiotics. If they still continue, you may need the doses of your immunosuppressant drugs (e.g. tacrolimus or ciclosporin) reduced.

Colds and 'flu
Colds and influenza (the 'flu) may also be more common after a transplant. People who have had a transplant may get these infections more frequently, or they may take longer than expected to recover after an infection. People who have had a transplant are recommended to take advantage of a free 'flu jab every year. These injections are generally safe after transplantation, but there have been reports of occasional side effects. So if you have ever had the 'flu jab before and felt unwell afterwards, please make sure you talk to your kidney doctor about it, and mention it to your GP as well. Some health centres offer 'flu jabs to carers and other people living with the transplant patient as well, as an added precaution.

Pneumonia
Pneumonia (a severe infection in the lungs) is rare after a transplant, but most hospitals give preventative treatment for six months after the operation. This treatment will stop you getting a rare infection called *Pneumocystis carinii*, which is caused by a germ that is common in the environment but only results in infection when the body's immune system is suppressed. The preventative treatment is one tablet of co-trimoxazole (Septrin) daily for six months after transplantation.

Cytomegalovirus (CMV)
There is one infection that is a particular problem after transplantation. It is called cytomegalovirus (CMV) infection. For most people who are not

taking immunosuppressant drugs, CMV is a mild infection that causes a 'flu-like illness. However, in patients who have just received a transplant, CMV infection can be quite a severe illness. The risk of developing CMV is highest in the three months following your transplant operation. This is because if you have ever had the virus it will lie dormant in your body for the rest of your life after the infection. Many kidneys that are donated for transplant contain hidden CMV, which can then 'wake up' to cause a new infection in the recipient. Testing to help you avoid CMV includes measurement of your own natural defences against the virus. If these defences are low, you may be given a course of tablets to prevent CMV for the first couple of months following the transplant.

Epstein-Barr virus (EBV)

EBV is the virus that causes glandular fever, an illness which usually affects adolescents or young adults. It makes them ill for a couple of weeks with fevers and swollen glands, often on the side of the neck. In people without kidney disease, the infection normally goes away and there is a full recovery, though some people do feel 'washed out' for several weeks after the infection. It is possible to get an infection with EBV after a kidney transplant. This is because someone who has had EBV will always have the virus in their body, even if it isn't causing any symptoms. It only causes problems if a person's defences against infection are reduced. Of course this is what happens when immunosuppressant drugs are given after a kidney transplant.

If EBV does develop, it usually happens within 6–12 weeks after the transplant operation. Symptoms include fevers and a loss of energy, similar to the symptoms of CMV (see above). EBV infection can be diagnosed with a blood test. If someone who has had a transplant does get EBV, it can usually be cured by reducing their dose of immunosuppressant drugs. Some units test all their transplant patients for EBV three months after the transplant, and may find a positive blood test even if someone is well. This is nothing to be worried about, but some doctors feel it may be a sign that the immunosuppressant drugs are causing too much suppression of the immune system, and will reduce the doses of these drugs.

In some cases, an EBV infection can cause very swollen glands in the body, and a condition called PTLD (a type of lymphoma or cancer of the lymph glands, see page 116) may develop. This is a serious condition, and requires urgent treatment. So if you have a transplant and your lymph glands become enlarged, especially if you have a slightly tender swelling on the sides of the neck, you should tell your transplant team. In most cases, the swelling will be caused by a minor viral infection or sore throat, but it is important the doctors check you for EBV and PTLD.

Chicken pox and shingles

Chicken pox is a virus that causes a disease where the skin breaks out in tiny blisters, often all over the body. When the blisters are fresh and leaking fluid, chicken pox is infectious. The blisters take a little while to heal fully, but once new blisters have stopped appearing, the risk of infection is reduced. Shingles is a skin infection in adults that is caused by the chicken pox virus, so someone with shingles and fresh blisters is also potentially infectious.

If you did not have chicken pox as a child, you won't have any natural resistance to this infection and so will be more prone to catching it. Chicken pox in someone who is taking immunosuppressant medication can be very serious, so it is important you avoid touching (or any other close contact with) children who have chicken pox. If contact does occur, telephone your transplant unit immediately. The doctors at your kidney unit will know whether any natural immunity to chicken pox has shown up in your blood tests. If you have this natural immunity, there is usually no need for special action. However, if you have no natural immunity, the transplant unit may give you an injection of globulin (anti-chicken pox antibody) straight away to reduce the chances of a severe infection.

It is helpful to ask the transplant centre what your natural immunity to chicken pox is, so that you know how to seek advice urgently if you do come into contact with someone who does have chicken pox or shingles.

Even if you don't come into contact with chicken pox, someone with a transplant can get shingles. Although shingles is caused by the same virus, it is a far less serious problem unless it affects the surface of the eye. Nevertheless, it does require urgent treatment.

BK virus

A virus called the BK virus has recently been discovered. If this does occur, it is usually quite soon after the operation when doses of immunosuppressant medication are at their highest. However, it can occasionally crop up later, even after a year.

BK virus can stop the transplanted kidney from functioning properly. A drug called cidofovir is used to treat this virus, although it is not yet known how effective it is. It is given as a course of injections.

PREVENTION OF INFECTION AFTER A TRANSPLANT

The prevention of infection after a transplant is important. You will be prescribed a number of drugs to prevent infection for the first 6 or 12 months after the transplant operation. Different transplant centres prescribe different combinations of drugs, but the most commonly used are:

- Co-trimoxazole to prevent *Pneumocystis* pneumonia;

- Amphotericin to prevent thrush in the mouth or gullet;

- Isoniazid to prevent tuberculosis (TB) in people who are have a high risk of this condition;

- Antibiotics to prevent urine infections. These are particularly useful for people who get a lot of urine infections.

Helping yourself

If you have had a transplant recently, there are many things you can do to prevent infections. For the first few months after the transplant operation, it might be a good idea to keep away (as far as possible) from people who have bad colds or 'flu. In the early days, when your doses of immuno-suppressants will be particularly high, warn your friends and relatives that they should keep away from you if they are at all unwell. Try to avoid travelling in close, crowded places such as on public transport. In the longer term, it is important you feel able to lead a normal life – that, after all, is why you opted to have the transplant in the first place. So, once you have made an initial recovery from surgery, it won't be necessary to keep away from everyone who is ill. You don't need to live in a bubble.

IF IT ALL GETS TOO MUCH

Receiving a kidney transplant is normally a happy event, giving you the prospect of a life free from dialysis. However, it is also a very stressful time. The transplant may not work immediately, or there may be problems such as rejection in the first few weeks, which give rise to worries over whether the transplant will fail or not. You may have very high expectations of a rapid recovery, but a transplant involves a major surgical operation. It takes most people three months to get back to normal after major surgery, even if they go home from hospital a week after the operation.

Coming to terms with the pace of recovery may be even more difficult for someone who receives a transplant before they start dialysis. If you are on dialysis, a transplant will almost always make you feel better as soon as it starts to function and dialysis is no longer needed. For someone who has not yet started dialysis, the transplant will almost certainly make you feel less well than you were beforehand. Of course, the transplant will be a good thing in the long term. But in the short term it can be a shock to be hospitalised, have a major operation, and then have to take many more tablets every day.

Even if someone has been on dialysis a long time, the prospect of a life without dialysis can be frightening. Obviously it is good not to need dialysis. But for people who have built their life's routine to accommodate dialysis, and have made good friends on the dialysis unit, it may be hard to be separated from this way of life. The whole routine of a life without dialysis will need to be rebuilt, and while this is exciting and a wonderful opportunity, it can also be very challenging.

So you will have to cope with some stress and emotional difficulties after the transplant, even if it goes very well. This can be hard to cope with, and some people find it hard to talk about the problems, because they think everyone else is expecting them to be pleased and grateful for the transplant. Sometimes people get depressed and find it difficult to take their tablets regularly or to come to clinic. Occasionally, the depression causes physical symptoms, or magnifies minor health problems in people's consciousness. This may mean the doctors end up performing many extra tests in case the symptoms are due to an underlying unusual infection or other medical problem.

Someone with a transplant who feels stressed or depressed may affect the people around them. This can be a problem if someone has received a kidney from a living donor – their donor may feel that they are being ungrateful. Donors can also suffer some depression immediately after the transplant and that adds more pressure.

It is best to anticipate some of these problems before the transplant, and discuss your hopes and fears with those close to you and with the transplant team. It is particularly helpful to talk to someone who has received a kidney transplant. His or her perspective will be rather different from those of the doctors, nurses and transplant coordinators. You may find it refreshing, and very helpful. In living donation this is particularly helpful as it allows both parties to compare problems. The medical team will usually have no idea what it's actually like (unless they are a donor or recipient themselves); however, they may have done or seen many hundreds of operations over the years.

If you find your mood is down after the transplant, don't bottle up your emotions or feel guilty about your feelings. Talk to someone who can offer you support – this may be someone close to you, the transplant nurse or doctor. People do come through a period of stress or depression after a transplant, but you cannot do it easily on your own. A few people benefit from a course of anti-depressant tablets, which can be taken safely in combination with the immunosuppressant drugs.

THREE MONTHS OUT, AND OK?

If you get to three months, you are out of hospital and well, with a creatinine of less than 200 µmol/L and you have not had any significant rejection, CMV or any other significant infection . . . congratulations. This is a good start. If transplantation is the Grand National, you are over the 'second hurdle', but you are not there yet. A good transplant is one that is working well at one year or more, not three months.

KEY FACTS

1. The two most common problems in the first 3 months are rejection and infection.

2. 'Rejection' is when the body sees the new kidney as a 'foreign body', and tries to get rid of it.

3. Rejection can be acute (short-term) or chronic (long-term).

4. Acute rejection happens rapidly, usually within the first 3 months after the operation.

5. If a patient stops taking their immunosuppressant drugs (even for a short period) they will get acute rejection.

6. Acute rejection is relatively easy to treat with a course of high dose steroids.

7. Chronic rejection happens over a much longer period of time.

8. Immunosuppressant drugs reduce the body's ability to fight infections

9 Many transplant patients will get an infection after the operation although it's not usually serious.

10 Transplant patients should try to stay away from people with infections such as colds or 'flu, especially in the first 3 months.

11 Transplant patients may develop diabetes after the operation, due to side effects of the drugs. This can require insulin.

10
Looking after yourself and your transplant over the years

This chapter explains what happens in the months and years after the operation. We discuss how to make sure that your kidney transplant lasts for as long as possible and that you remain fit and healthy.

Looking after your transplanted kidney for the long term is just as important as looking after it in the early days. Make a *real effort* every day, no matter whether it is the 5th or 15th anniversary of your kidney. To make sure that your new kidney lasts for as long as possible, it is important to take all your prescribed medications, attend clinics and look after your general health. This might sound easy to do, but it can be very hard. There are a great many medications to take, and they can have unpleasant side effects. Hospital clinics may be inconvenient and, if your clinic visits mean going back to the unit where you used to go for haemodialysis, this can bring back painful memories. On the other hand, if you have been using a home treatment (such as peritoneal dialysis) frequent trips to hospital can be a real shock to your system.

Keeping your transplant kidney healthy means making an effort **every single day**, not just 'when you remember'! Try to keep these points in mind:

- Not all kidney patients are lucky enough to get a transplant.

- There are lots of things that you can do to make sure that your kidney stays healthy today, such as taking your medication and keeping fit and well.

- If you feel ill, you should contact your transplant team immediately. You will need to be checked out and will probably need a blood test.

But if you stop looking after your transplant, even for a short period of time, your body may well seize its chance to reject your new kidney. Many transplants fail simply because people don't take their medications properly, or miss their clinic appointments. Don't let this happen to you.

Depending on where you live, you are likely to receive long-term care for your kidney transplant from your local kidney unit, rather than from the centre where the transplant was performed. Usually, this will be so that treatment can be given nearer your home. The consultant responsible for your care will be either the consultant you saw when you were on dialysis, or one who specialises in transplantation. If you would prefer, however, you can choose to have your long-term care at the transplant centre, even if that means travelling further. If this is what feels right for you, ask your transplant team if that is possible.

There are two ways that you can help yourself: stay in touch and take control.

STAY IN TOUCH

It is very important to know the best ways to contact all the people who look after you. This could be with a direct telephone line (phoning the hospital switchboard isn't usually very quick or effective), or by email. Renal units might differ in the way that they prefer to be contacted, so it's best to check with your transplant team which number or email address they recommend you use.

The people for whom you really must have contact details are:

- Your consultant kidney doctor;

- Your transplant coordinator;

- Your transplant nurse;

- Your dietitian;

- Your renal pharmacist;

- The clinic (in case you need to change an appointment);

- The place where you can get more of the specialist drugs if you run out. This is particularly important for your immunosuppressants.

You should also know who to get in touch with if there is an urgent problem and you need to be seen the same day. Realising you have forgotten to take your immunosuppressants for more than 24 hours, or vomiting and not being able to keep your tablets down are both examples of urgent problems. So is any infection that causes your temperature to go above 38°, or any severe urine infection – especially if you have pain over the transplant, or blood in your urine.

If any of these occur, you need to see a transplant nurse or doctor as soon as possible. There are several ways. The simplest is to go to the ward on your kidney unit. It may be better to ring the hospital and ask to speak to the consultant on call or kidney registrar (middle grade doctor), and then take their advice. If you decide to go to Accident and Emergency, make it clear you are a kidney patient, and need to see a specialist doctor or nurse. (The doctors in A&E are often junior, with limited knowledge of kidney medicine.)

TAKE CONTROL

It is very sensible to learn as much as you can about your blood results. Many units have signed up to a service that enables patients to see their blood results through a secure server on the Internet (the Renal-PatientView website, see Appendix 1). You can also ask to have copies of the letters written to your GP after you attend transplant clinic appointments. Some units do this routinely. Your relationship with your GP is important too. GPs may not be experts on transplantation, but you will find they know more than hospital specialists about many other conditions. And it will be your GP who prescribes most or all of your medication. Good relationships with your local pharmacy are very useful, especially when it comes to queries or repeat prescriptions.

When you talk to anyone about medication or medical needs always start by saying: 'I am a transplant patient'. It can help enormously and prevent many problems.

Know your disease – keep information

As you are reading this book, it is safe to assume that you want to know more. So, in a way, we are preaching to the converted. Of course, reading it will not necessarily mean that you follow all the advice in the book, or read it all.

Nonetheless, there are other things you can do to stay in control. Why not keep a file, or folder, of all your information? Keep a notebook, and when you have dealings with any doctor, GP or hospital, write down their name, how to contact them, and what decisions were made during that interaction. Keep a list of the things that are important such as an up-to-date list of your drugs, your latest blood tests, copies of clinic letters as you get them and anything else that you think may help you and others to remain in control of your treatment.

CHRONIC REJECTION
(OR CHRONIC ALLOGRAFT NEPHROPATHY)

'Chronic' means long term and slow starting. It does not necessarily require immediate action. Some doctors think that the term 'chronic rejection' is misleading. Chronic rejection is very different from acute rejection, in that the immune system does not attack and reject the transplant kidney in the same way as it does in acute rejection. The immune system may start a process of damage, but slow scarring that occurs inside the transplanted kidney depends on factors such as high blood pressure. This is why some doctors call the process 'chronic allograft nephropathy' rather than 'rejection'.

Chronic rejection is more like a slow ageing of the new kidney. The cause is uncertain. If it happens, it will usually start more than a year after the transplant operation. Doctors may suspect chronic rejection if a patient's blood creatinine starts to rise slowly after it has been stable for some time. Alternatively, an increasing amount of protein in the urine may be the first sign of chronic rejection. This can lead to ankle swelling. More often than not, you cannot tell the process has started, or whether it is getting better, or not. As with acute rejection (see above), the only sure way to diagnose the condition is to do a biopsy.

The severity of chronic rejection varies. Mild chronic rejection is not usually a problem. However, more severe chronic rejection will eventually cause the new kidney to fail. When this happens the person will need to go back to dialysis or have another transplant. Chronic rejection may take years to happen, but it is the most common cause of transplant failure after the first year.

The treatment of chronic rejection includes adjusting the immunosuppressant drugs. Some of these drugs can be harmful to the kidney and adjusting the dose or changing to an alternative drug can reduce this. It is also important to keep the blood pressure well controlled, and make sure it doesn't go too high.

In addition to staying in touch and looking after yourself, you should be aware of some of the problems that may occur following a kidney transplant and how they may be prevented or treated.

LOOKING AFTER YOURSELF

After you have had a kidney transplant, you should work with your doctor to:

- Keep your blood pressure down (under 140/90 mmHg; or 130/80 mmHg if you are taking blood pressure drugs). This is probably the most important thing you can do for yourself.

- To do this, monitor your own blood pressure twice a week, between appointments. This is not expensive (you can buy a machine from a high street pharmacy for around £10–15). An added advantage of checking your blood pressure yourself is that it can often be raised simply by being in a hospital environment ('white coat syndrome').

- Keep your weight at an appropriate level and eat a balanced diet.

- Stop smoking.

- Take regular exercise.

- Keep your diabetes (if you have it) under control.

- Try to spot the onset of diabetes, if you did not have it before the transplant. If you think you might be at risk of getting diabetes, ask your transplant doctor to review the drugs that you are taking. Some of them might need to be changed.

- Keep your cholesterol low.

- Having your blood thinned by taking a small dose of aspirin is likely to be appropriate in your case.

- If you are on prednisolone, have your bone density checked regularly.

- Make sure you have your annual 'flu and pneumonia injections.

- Look after your skin by avoiding sunlight and looking for new moles or lumps. Ask a doctor to look over all of your skin, at least once a year.

CIRCULATION PROBLEMS AND HIGH BLOOD PRESSURE

What are circulation problems?

About 30% (just under a third) of the population of the UK will develop serious circulation problems. However, people who have had a kidney transplant are 20 times more likely to get these problems than people who have not had one. People who have diabetes are also at increased risk of circulation problems.

The circulation consists of the blood vessels all around the body. The blood vessels that come out of the heart to supply the body, called the arteries, are under particular strain because a lot of blood flows through them. The walls of the arteries are stretched and put under pressure each time the heart beats.

Over many years, this stress can lead to damage to the arteries, which occurs much faster if the blood pressure is high or if there is too much fat (particularly one type of fat called cholesterol) in the blood. Damaged arteries can cause disease in all parts of the body, most particularly in the heart itself (a heart attack), in the neck and brain (causing stroke), or in the legs (gangrene). Damaged arteries can also cause disease inside the kidney transplant.

Prevention of circulation problems

There are several important things that can be done to reduce the risk of circulation problems after a transplant. If you smoke, far and away the most important thing you can do is to stop. This can be difficult because nicotine is very addictive, but nicotine patches, hypnotism or acupuncture can all help you to give up. NHS 'Stop Smoking' advice can be helpful too.

A healthy diet and regular exercise will help, as will making sure that your weight does not go up too much after a transplant.

High blood pressure

Blood flows around the body under pressure generated by the pumping action of the heart. The blood pressure varies from minute to minute, and is meant to rise to high levels under strenuous exercise.

However, in many people with kidney problems, the blood pressure remains high all the time. This is a particular problem after a transplant, and at least half of transplant recipients have high blood pressure, usually with no symptoms.

Two numbers measure blood pressure. One of these numbers is the highest pressure of blood as the heart pumps blood out (known as the systolic blood pressure). The other number is the lowest pressure of the blood, in between heartbeats (the diastolic blood pressure). The Renal Association (the society for British kidney doctors) recommends that the blood pressure of someone who has a kidney transplant should ideally be lower than 130/80 mmHg. The doctors in the transplant unit will make sure that each individual patient has medicines that give them the best possible blood pressure so that the risks of damage from high blood pressure will be reduced.

Some people cannot get their blood pressure down to the recommended low levels, despite taking several types of drug. This may be because drugs cause side effects, or because there is some hardening of the arteries in the blood and a higher blood pressure is required to get blood around the body. It could also be because the blood pressure can be higher when it's measured in clinic than it is in day-to-day life (sometimes called the 'white coat effect'). It is likely that this is because going to see the doctor, or being in hospital, is a stressful experience for many people.

CHOLESTEROL

Cholesterol is a fatty substance, and is one of several different types of fat found in the body. It has several very important functions and is carried around in the blood. If blood vessels are damaged, however, cholesterol can become stuck to the inside, eventually causing narrowing. This is more likely to occur if the blood level of cholesterol is high, which depends on several factors. A tendency to high cholesterol may run in families. A diet high in fat may lead to a high cholesterol level. Also, high levels of protein in your urine, sometimes due to chronic rejection, can worsen high blood pressure and cholesterol levels.

The ideal cholesterol level

Research shows that low cholesterol levels can help to keep the transplant kidney healthy. The medical advice about ideal cholesterol levels is changing in line with ongoing research. The Renal Association has recommended that people with kidney disease who are at risk of disease in their circulation should have a cholesterol level of less than 5.0 mmol/L, and there is a more recent European recommendation of less than 4.5 mmol/L. Research in people without kidney disease has suggested that someone who is known to have disease in their circulation (heart attacks and strokes) should have a total cholesterol of less than 4.0 mmol/L.

Diet for reducing cholesterol

Foods that are high in cholesterol include dairy products, eggs and the fatty parts of red meat. Many processed foods can contain a lot of cholesterol and you should check the information on the labels carefully. The type of fats that increase blood cholesterol levels are often called 'saturated fats', while 'unsaturated fats' (such as olive oil) may be less harmful. The aim with diet is to reduce the amount of harmful fats that you eat, and to maintain a balanced diet with the right amounts of protein, carbohydrate, and fresh fruit and vegetables.

Drugs to reduce cholesterol

If diet and losing weight do not bring the blood cholesterol down to acceptable levels, drugs may be used. The type of drug most often used is called a 'statin'. Statins stop the body from making cholesterol in the liver. There are several different types of statin drugs, and if your doctor thinks you need this type of treatment, he or she will look for the one that is likely to suit you best. The decision will also depend on guidelines produced by your local health authority.

Any drug can have side effects in some people, and statins are no exception. Some people feel generally unwell with nausea or sickness as a result of taking a statin, and may have to stop the drug if this persists. Statins can cause aches and pains in the muscles. This is a serious side effect and if it happens to you, you should tell your doctor immediately.

WHO SHOULD HAVE CHOLESTEROL-LOWERING DRUGS?

Unfortunately, doctors don't know for certain when to recommend statins to people with kidney transplants. They have been proven to reduce the risk of heart attacks and strokes in people without kidney disease, but those with severe kidney disease were not included in most previous research, though trials are now under way.

Because of this uncertainty, doctors may make different recommendations according to their point of view. Some believe that statins must give similar protection to everyone and use them just as they would in people without kidney disease. Others believe that everyone who has a kidney transplant should be given statins, because their risk of heart attack and stroke is higher than in the general population. A further group believes that the decision should be based on the individual's cholesterol level.

As well as the drugs described above, which help lower cholesterol and blood pressure, many transplant patients are also prescribed one small aspirin tablet a day. This thins the blood and reduces the chances of arteries blocking.

Not everyone who has had a transplant will have to take all of these drugs. It is important to ask your doctor which ones you are taking and why you are not being prescribed others.

Lifestyle changes for blood pressure and circulation problems

Making changes to your lifestyle can reduce cholesterol and lower your blood pressure. There are also drugs that can be prescribed to help. The lifestyle changes that can be made include taking regular exercise and stopping smoking. It is also important to eat a healthy diet with lots of fresh fruit and vegetables, and without too much salt or fat.

Many transplant patients will also have to take a number of medicines to help lower their blood pressure and/or cholesterol. Many of these drugs have side effects, so if a new tablet causes problems, it is essential that you tell your doctor straight away. An alternative can usually be found.

DIABETES

The normal blood sugar level is between 3 and 7 mmol/L. If the blood sugar level (when taken at any time of the day) is over 11 mmol/L, or a fasting level (done in the morning, before having anything to eat) is over 7 mmol/L, then you have diabetes.

Diabetes is one of the most common causes of kidney failure, so it may be the reason why many people with diabetes have received, or are considering, a kidney transplant. But diabetes can also develop as a side effect of many immunosuppressant drugs including prednisolone, ciclosporin and tacrolimus. Depending on the drug regime, 5–15% of patients, who did not have diabetes before the transplant, will develop it.

Your risk of developing diabetes will be greater after a kidney transplant if you are from a non-Caucasian ethnic group, particularly if you are black or south Asian. If other members of your family have diabetes already, your risk of developing it will also be high.

Diagnosis of diabetes after a transplant

If you are going to develop diabetes after receiving a transplant, it is most likely to happen within the first three months. Everyone who has a transplant will have a routine blood test to measure their blood sugar levels before and after the operation, with regular repeat tests during the first few months. Ask what your blood sugar is every time you have a blood test. The fasting level should be less than 7 mmol/L. Having regular blood tests will mean that any changes in the blood sugar level can be detected *before* you get symptoms.

The symptoms of diabetes are:

- Thirst;

- Passing urine frequently;

- Infections such as thrush (an infection causing a sore throat or itching in the genital area).

If you find you have any of these symptoms after your transplant operation, you should ask your kidney doctor or specialist nurse to check for diabetes.

Some people who already have diabetes (usually Type 1 diabetes, which means they have to take insulin every day) have the opportunity to have a double kidney and pancreas transplant. The organs have to be taken from a deceased donor, because a living donor needs his or her own pancreas, so there are not as many options available as there are for straightforward kidney transplants. But those who are fortunate enough to be offered a kidney and a pancreas (both of which will come from the same deceased donor) can look forward not only to freedom from dialysis after the transplant, but freedom from the problems of diabetes as well. Dialysis can stop, and so can insulin injections. Not all transplant units do kidney and pancreas transplants, however. You may have to be referred to a specialist transplant centre, which could be a long way from your home.

CAN DIABETES AFTER A TRANSPLANT BE PREVENTED?

Some of the drugs given to keep the transplant working – the immuno-suppressant drugs – can cause diabetes as a side effect. The steroid drug prednisolone can cause diabetes, as can ciclosporin and tacrolimus. These drugs are vital in preventing the body from rejecting the transplant kidney so, unfortunately, at the moment there aren't any alternatives.

Even if one of these drugs does cause diabetes, it is usually not possible to stop taking it completely.

Tacrolimus causes diabetes in about 15% of patients. Ciclosporin causes diabetes in only about 5% of patients. Tacrolimus, however, is often better at preventing rejection. The actual risk is higher than this, as other drugs (such as prednisolone) can also cause diabetes. Older patients, and non-Caucasian patients, are also at increased risk whichever drug is used.

Anyone who has had a transplant should be monitored regularly for the signs of diabetes. If it's spotted early by your doctors, and (if you are taking tacrolimus) a quick switch to ciclosporin can be made, it might be possible to prevent full-blown diabetes from developing.

Sadly, it is not usually spotted in time. You could try to spot it yourself by watching your blood glucose very closely (at least 2–3 times a week) in the first three months after a transplant, then tell your doctors if your fasting blood sugar rises to higher than 7 mmol/L, more than once. Ask your transplant nurse what is the best way for you to do this.

Problems caused by diabetes

Diabetes is a disease that causes the level of sugar in the blood to become unstable, initially with a high level. Sugar is needed for energy by all parts of the body, and sugar is dissolved in the blood so that it can be carried around. The level of sugar in the blood usually stays the same throughout the day. If you eat a lot of sugar, for example a chocolate bar, the sugar passes into your body very quickly and the levels of sugar in your blood go up. An organ in the body called the pancreas releases a hormone called insulin when blood sugar levels are high. Insulin makes sure that any excess sugar in the blood is taken into storage.

If you do not eat all day and your blood sugar levels are low, your pancreas will stop producing insulin. Sugar will be released from storage, so that the level of sugar in your blood goes back up to normal levels.

If you have diabetes, your pancreas won't work as it should, so the sugar levels in your blood will not be properly controlled. You will need to reuce the amount of sugar in your diet and either take medication or inject yourself with insulin on a regular basis to make sure that your blood sugar levels don't go too high. If you do not eat for a long time, the level of sugar in your blood will fall too low, and you will need to eat immediately.

Diabetes can cause problems in the short term (blood sugar problems) and in the long term (infection and circulation problems).

High and low blood sugar levels

If you have too much sugar in your blood ('hyperglycaemia'), some sugar will pass through your kidneys into the urine. This in turn makes your kidney pass more urine, leading to a shortage of water in your body which will make you thirsty. If you have had a transplant, this process can cause your new kidney to function less well.

If your blood sugar level is very high, you can feel sick (or even vomit), have difficulty breathing, and in time you can fall into a coma if it is left unchecked.

Monitoring your own blood glucose is not complicated with the new machines that are available. If you have diabetes, your diabetes nurse will teach you how to do this and will also tell you how often you should self-monitor.

Low sugar levels in your blood starve the brain of the sugar it needs for energy, leading to slurred speech and a feeling of disorientation, as though you had had too much alcohol. Eventually, you may become unconscious ('hypoglycaemic coma'). Someone who is in hypoglycaemic coma (often called a 'hypo' for short) is at risk of having fits or even dying. Hypos must be treated urgently with a sugary drink or an injection of glucose. If the person is unconscious, you should call an ambulance. They will need an injection of glucagon or something sweet (glucose gel or honey) rubbed onto their gums while you are waiting for the paramedics. However, prevention is always better than a cure. Eating regular meals and taking the drugs given for diabetes will make you much less likely to have hypos.

Infection and circulation problems

If a person's blood sugar level is too high, they may not feel any different, but hidden damage is taking place. The body's defences do not work properly when the sugar levels are too high, so the body is at more risk of infection. These infections might be minor such as urine infections or skin infections, but more serious infections such as pneumonia or septicaemia (infection in the blood) can occur.

High sugar levels over a period of years can make circulation problems much worse. This is because diabetes speeds up the process of hardening of the arteries (atherosclerosis or arterial narrowing). Heart attack, stroke or problems due to poor circulation to the legs can also develop.

Diabetes can affect your eyes as well. Eye problems caused by diabetes can take some time to develop. They are most common in people who had diabetes before having a transplant. You should have the back of your eyes checked once a year with an instrument called an ophthalmoscope (it is the same size as a torch with a bright light shining out of the side at the top). This can be done by your optician, or eye specialist (ophthalmologist) at the hospital. There is an NHS screening programme for patients who might be at risk, which means that you should be called regularly (via your GP) for eye screening. You can usually be seen reasonably close to where you live.

If diabetic eye disease is detected, you should be considered for treatment, possibly including laser treatment to the back of the eye, the retina. It is very important to have these eye checks so that any damage can be minimised or even prevented. There is a risk that the damage can cause blindness if it isn't monitored and treated.

Treatment of diabetes

The aim of treatment for diabetes is to keep the levels of sugar in the blood close to normal all the time. There is a special blood test called an HbA_{1c}. This reflects the control of diabetes over the last three months, the lower the number the better. The aim is to keep it under 7%.

How can you do this? It is very important to control the amount of sugar you eat.

Being overweight makes diabetes much worse. Whether or not you have had a kidney transplant, carrying too much fat significantly increases your risk of developing diabetes in the first place. So it is important to lose weight if you are overweight, and to avoid putting on weight if you are not. Losing weight can be difficult but, for some people who are developing diabetes, it can be all that is needed to make it go away completely.

A healthy diet is all that some people with diabetes need for their treatment. However many people will also need to take drugs as well. These drugs are either tablets to lower their blood sugar, or injections of insulin. Insulin is the body's natural substance for regulating the amount of sugar in the blood; boosting the level of insulin after meals with an injection may be needed to keep the sugar levels stable.

More information about diabetes is available from Diabetes UK (see Appendix 2 for full details).

CANCER

Immunosuppressant drugs are given to transplant patients to prevent the body's immune system from rejecting the new kidney. They work by making the immune system less efficient. However, one of the functions of the immune system is to fight cancer. Because transplant patients have a weakened immune system, they are at greater risk of developing cancer than they would have been before the operation. A research study has shown that a quarter of all transplant patients who live for 25 years after a transplant develop some type of cancer.

Skin cancers

Transplant patients are far more likely than other people to get skin cancer. This makes it very important for people who have had a transplant to use a strong 'sun block' cream to avoid exposure to the sun; the risk depends on sun *exposure*, just avoiding sunburn is not enough. Use at least a factor 35 sun cream – higher if you can find it. Factor 60 or even 75 is available if you look (see pages 124–5 for more details on avoiding the harmful effects of the sun). Exposure to the sun greatly increases the risk of developing skin cancer. The risk also depends on skin colour. The people at highest risk are those with fair hair, blue eyes and fair skin. People of Asian or black race have a much lower risk of developing skin cancer.

In northern Australia, where skin cancer is particularly common, the increased risk to transplant patients rises so that one out of every three transplant patients will develop skin cancer unless they take extreme precautions. In the UK, one in 10 people who have had a kidney transplant for 10 years will have had a skin cancer.

You should be aware of the chance of getting skin cancer, and keep an eye out for any new dark spots, moles or lesions on your skin. Skin cancer may also occur on the back, so someone else will need to check there. As well as skin cancers, you are also more likely to develop warts on the skin, and it can be hard to tell the difference between a wart and a skin cancer. Signs of skin cancer include an abnormality that is growing fast, bleeds, or is raised but has a crater in the middle. It is better to be safe than sorry, so any skin abnormality giving cause for concern should be checked by a doctor. If someone has had a skin cancer, they are at risk of getting more and should be seen routinely in a specialist skin clinic. Also, if you have had a skin cancer, you should have the prescription for your immuno-suppressant drugs reviewed, to see if the dosage should be reduced or the type of drugs changed.

Some renal units are even more careful than this, and arrange for a skin specialist (dermatologist) to look over your whole body for cancers and pre-cancers, once a year. This is particularly important if you have already had a skin cancer, as the chances of developing another one are high.

Provided that skin cancers are diagnosed in good time, they are not usually life threatening. Skin cancer does not usually spread to other parts of the body, and can be easily removed in most cases, though a larger lesion may need specialist plastic surgery and a skin graft – that is one reason why spotting the cancers early helps the treatment.

Lymphoma (PTLD)

Between 2 and 5% of people who have a kidney transplant develop a type pf lymphoma called 'post transplant lymphoproliferative disease' (PTLD for short), often *within a year* of the operation. This is a serious leukaemia-like cancer of the bone marrow and immune system. It is more common in people who have had stronger immunosuppressant drugs. It is often caused by Epstein-Barr Virus (see page 96), however most people who get

JOHN'S DILEMMA: LYMPHOMA OR DIALYSIS?

John was delighted to get his kidney transplant. He was 60 years old when he got kidney failure. Then he spent 6 years on CAPD, so he felt he had 'done his time'. The kidney worked well from the start and he had no problems with rejection or infections. But three months after the transplant, lumps started appearing on both sides of his neck. At first he ignored them, thinking they would go away. When they didn't, he showed them to his transplant nurse, who made sure he was admitted immediately to hospital for a CT scan of his chest and tummy, and a biopsy of one of the lumps. He couldn't understand what the fuss was about. He was then sent home. He cried all night, as he knew something was up, but no one would tell him what they suspected.

The next day he was summoned to the transplant clinic, where a doctor he didn't know told him he had lymphoma, a type of cancer, related to the immunosuppressant drugs he was taking. John couldn't believe it. After the initial shock, he met his consultant two days later, who said it was not necessarily a fatal type of cancer. She explained that by stopping most of immunosuppressant drugs (risking rejection), the cancer may melt away.

After six months, and several more scans, he was told that the lymphoma was 'going away'. And slowly the doses of all his immunosuppressant tablets were increased. Fortunately the kidney did not reject. He couldn't think what would be worse: losing the kidney through rejection, and returning to dialysis (and knowing that he would be unlikely to get another kidney) or dying of lymphoma. He feels his neck every day. So far, the lymphoma has not come back.

EBV after a transplant do not get PTLD. PTLD is a life threatening condition and can lead to death in about 40% of people who get it, though treatments are improving all the time.

It can be very dangerous to stop taking immunosuppressant drugs under normal circumstances. However if a patient does get lymphoma, it may be their only hope of recovery. If the doctors do decide to stop your immunosuppressant drugs to try to cure lymphoma, they will keep a very close eye on your transplant kidney to make sure that it doesn't stop working. There may be situations where stopping the immunosuppressant drugs does cause the kidney to fail and the patient will have to start dialysis treatment again. Although this would be very distressing, it might be preferable to dying of lymphoma.

In some cases chemotherapy drugs are needed to treat lymphoma. If you do develop lymphoma or PTLD, your transplant team and the lymphoma specialists will discuss the most appropriate treatment for you in detail.

Other cancers

Other types of cancer are more common after a kidney transplant than in the general population. Women have an increased risk of cancer of the cervix (neck of the womb), mostly because this cancer is caused by a viral infection of the cervix. This type of cancer is preventable if cervical smears are performed regularly in women who are sexually active. There are no national guidelines for cervical smear testing in transplant patients in the UK, but many units advise sexually active women to have an annual smear – more frequent than the three-yearly smears advised in the national screening programme.

Some cancers in other parts of the body are at least twice as common in people with a kidney transplant as in the general population. This includes bowel, lung and breast cancer. Therefore it is even more important that if you have a kidney transplant and smoke, that you stop. Also remember to take part in screening tests for breast and bowel cancer that you may be asked to participate in as part of the general population screening.

PROBLEMS WITH YOUR BONES

Bones can become damaged while people are on dialysis, and one advantage of a transplant is that dialysis-related bone disease (called dialysis amyloidosis) can be prevented. However, there are other problems that can develop with the bones and joints following a transplant.

The biggest problem with the bones is osteoporosis. Osteoporosis is loss of strength of bone, making it more brittle. This loss of strength causes no pain or other symptoms, until the bones give way, with either a fracture of the arm or leg, or collapse and loss of height of one of the back-bones, usually in the lower back. All of these fractures will be painful. A fracture at the top of the femur (thigh bone), as it sits in the hip joint, is particularly common.

Because osteoporosis may cause no symptoms until a serious problem has occurred, many transplant units check all their patients for osteoporosis. Other units will perform checks if someone has had a fractured bone, especially if this is a 'low impact' fracture. There are several reasons why you might be at risk of osteoporosis after a kidney transplant. It could have developed while you were on dialysis, and is more likely to occur if you have diabetes. Steroid (prednisolone) treatment increases the risk of osteoporosis, and is often given after the transplant, and some people have been given steroids to treat their original kidney disease even before they started dialysis. There is also some loss of bone strength in the first few months after a transplant, when you are in hospital and generally less active. The loss of bone strength is much slower after this early period.

The scan for osteoporosis is a bone density scan, called a DEXA scan. It is like having an ordinary X-ray of the hip and spine, but the machine measures the exact density of your bones and compares it to normal levels for your age. About 50% of the people with kidney transplants have normal bone density, about 40% have slightly reduced bone density (called osteopenia), and 10% have osteoporosis. If you have osteopenia or osteoporosis, the treatment options should be discussed with your doctors. Osteopenia may not need any specific treatment if you have not had any fractures. Treatment options include reducing or stopping your steroid medication, though the benefit of this has to be balanced against any risk of reduced transplant function. There are drugs called biphosphonates which strengthen the bones, and most people with kidney transplants who have osteoporosis should take these. There are several similar drugs in this group; two of the ones commonly used are called risedronate and alendronate.

Other problems with the bones and joints include arthritis. This may occur in the knees, hips, spine or hands. Pain in these areas should not be confused with osteoporosis, which does not cause pain until the bone has given way. Arthritis pain can be treated with paracetamol. Drugs called NSAIDs (non-steroidal anti-inflammatory drugs) are commonly used to treat arthritic pain. They include aspirin and ibuprofen. Both of these drugs can be bought over the counter in pharmacies, or in supermarkets. You should **not** use NSAID drugs if you have a kidney transplant, unless you have specifically checked with your transplant specialist. Brand names for ibuprofen include Advil, Brufen and Nurofen. Other NSAIDs that can be prescribed by a doctor include diclofenac (often under the brand name Voltarol). All of these drugs can cause a reduction in the function of the transplant. Occasionally even one single dose can stop a kidney from working. If you have a transplant with very good function it may be safe to take some ibuprofen occasionally if you are not dehydrated at the time and do not have an infection of any sort, but do check with your transplant doctor first.

WARNING!

Do not use NSAIDs if you have a kidney transplant unless your kidney consultant says you can.

Common NSAIDs are:

- Aspirin [NB: low doses of aspirin to help thin the blood might be prescribed]
- Ibuprofen
- Advil
- Brufen
- Nurofen
- Diclofenac or Voltarol

DON'T buy over the counter medications without first telling the pharmacist you have a kidney transplant.

For people with severe arthritis, a knee or hip replacement may be the best treatment. If you have a kidney transplant, the risks of this major surgery are higher than for someone without kidney disease, but it is usually possible to perform joint replacement surgery safely in people with transplants. Certainly it should not be necessary to be immobile or in severe pain if you are otherwise fit for an operation. If surgery does take place, the orthopaedic team and the transplant team should work together to look after you, and the transplant doctors should keep an eye on you while you are in hospital.

KEY FACTS

1. Keeping your transplant kidney healthy means making an effort every single day.

2. Keep in touch with the renal unit and let them know as soon as you have a problem.

3. Take control by trying to learn as much as you can about your treatment.

4. Look after yourself – try to keep your blood pressure down, eat a healthy diet, take regular exercise and don't smoke.

5. Attending clinic regularly will enable the doctors to detect early signs of chronic rejection.

6. Chronic rejection can be treated by changing your immunosuppressant drugs.

7. Transplant patients can get circulation or blood pressure problems, often caused by high cholesterol levels in the blood.

8. Cancer is another side effect of immunosuppressant drugs.

9. The most common cancers to affect transplant patients are skin cancer and lymphoma (cancer of the lymph glands).

11
Living with your transplant

This chapter looks at some of the issues that will be with you in the long term when you have a transplant and explores how you can live a normal and enjoyable life as far as possible.

Once you have had your transplant and become used to your regime of regular check-ups and daily medication, your life may seem more 'normal' than it has done for years. No more dialysis sessions, no more PD exchanges in the car or corners of the office. No more making sure that the hospital can contact you, 24 hours a day, 365 days a year – just in case. You are likely to feel much better in yourself as well, and have more energy for enjoying life. So it is time to enjoy life again.

SOCIAL LIFE

If you have been used to organising your life round haemodialysis sessions, especially if these happened in hospital, you may find your new-found freedom exhilarating, scary or a mixture of both. Certainly, if you have a well-functioning transplant, you can pick up a 'normal' social life again in many respects. But there are a few golden rules that you should always remember:

❶ Take your tablets regularly, and without fail. If you are going away overnight or for a weekend, always take spares in case you are late back for any reason.

❷ Being on immunosuppressant medication will mean that you will be more vulnerable to infections than other people, so do avoid visiting friends if there is sickness in the house – particularly infectious diseases common among children such as diarrhoea and vomiting or chicken pox (see page 97).

❸ Be sensible about your own limits. None of us can party as hard at 50 as we could at 20. If you feel you have missed out on an exciting social life for several years due to being on dialysis, then you might be tempted to rush out and make up for lost time. But be gentle with yourself and don't get overtired.

On the other hand, your new kidney gives you a real opportunity to 'get your life back'. Enjoy it!

BACK TO WORK

If you have been on dialysis for some time, it may have been difficult for you to continue working. If this is the case, you may now be thinking about how to get back into the workplace. If your kidney unit has a social worker on the staff, a good place to begin is by talking to him or her. If you have been out of work for a while, however, you may find it better to begin by taking a part-time job if you can find one. If you are unused to working, you will find it tiring at first, but as you get used to the new routines, this should get easier.

Some people find that having been away from the workplace for a number of years leaves them with a blank CV, which can be difficult to explain to future employers. Try to be positive about this. Draw upon the experiences you have gained through being on dialysis to promote yourself. You might be able to get access to a college course or evening classes to help get back to work. It's important to be realistic and not expect too much all at once.

If you were only on dialysis for a short time, were on a home-based dialysis, or hadn't started dialysis (if you had a living donor transplant), you may still have an established position at work. You will, of course, need to take time off for the operation, but the time needed (3–6 months) would be similar for any other major surgery, and much of this is not planned. If you are in work, certain employment and sick pay rights will be assured. Do make sure you speak to someone in occupational health or human resources if you want to know what your employers are (and should be) offering you.

Smaller employers are sometimes the least sympathetic. Time off can become a problem, with statutory sick pay only being available. So it is important to ensure you have as much financial back-up as possible.

If you feel your employers are not treating you fairly, you should talk to your union representative if you have one, make an appointment at your local citizens' advice bureau, or ring the NKF Helpline.

HUGH: WHAT'S IMPORTANT – WORK OR HEALTH?

Hugh was a bit of a workaholic. He set up his own (catering) company when he was 22 years old and worked very hard to build it up over the next 20 years. He opened new branches every year. It was moving from strength to strength and he was constantly looking for opportunities to expand. He and his wife Sheila had two children, but she always felt that he didn't spend enough time at home as he was too obsessed with the company. The last thing he expected at the age of 42 was kidney failure. He went from feeling normal to needing peritoneal dialysis within four weeks.

Hugh mastered APD (which he thought was the best treatment for him to keeping working), and kept working though never felt completely well. When he came home he slept, or scratched himself all night and slept when he could.

Sheila immediately offered him one of her kidneys. After a three month work-up, Hugh had the transplant and it worked well. Sheila joked that it was as much for her sanity, as his health. Six months later, they treated themselves to a one week holiday in the Caribbean. After a long chat about what was important in life, Hugh came home, sold his beloved company, and is doing some voluntary work. He has never felt better, and Sheila says they have never been closer. In some ways, Hugh is glad he went into kidney failure, as it has given him an opportunity to reassess his life.

HOLIDAYS

Drugs to take when travelling

One of the advantages of having a successful kidney transplant is that it is much easier to travel than when you are on dialysis, so holidays are important to most patients with transplants. When travelling to some parts of the world there is an increased risk of some infections, and it may be advisable to take preventative medication (for example, against malaria), or have vaccinations.

For someone with a transplant, taking the right preventative treatment is important. Check with your kidney unit and travel company what preventative measures are advised, and then double check that the treatment is safe to take for someone with a transplant (see the NKF website for more detailed information).

Some people who are prone to developing urine infections may find it helpful to take a short course of antibiotics with them, so that they can start treatment at the first signs of a problem, avoiding the delays that might occur when finding a doctor who is confident to treat someone with a kidney transplant.

Vaccinations

Vaccination is a difficult issue after a transplant, mainly because vaccinations work by stimulating the immune system. When you have had a transplant, the immunosuppressant drugs suppress your immune system to prevent your body rejecting the new kidney, and so giving vaccinations can be risky. Many vaccines are safe, however, and can be given. Although problems are rare, they can happen. It is important, therefore, to be closely monitored if and when you do have a vaccination. There are some types of vaccines, such as 'live vaccines' e.g. MMR and Typhoid, which can never be given. Before having any type of vaccination, it is best to check with your travel service or a website resource such as the Hospital for Tropical Diseases in London. Then double check via the transplant team or the NKF whether the recommended treatments are safe. There is also more information available on the NKF website (see Appendix 2).

Don't forget your immunosuppressants

It is important to continue taking your immunosuppressant tablets without a break. So, if you are travelling, take more with you than you need in case something happens to delay your return journey.

It is important to plan ahead if you are travelling across time zones. It's a good idea to take one dose either a few hours earlier or a few hours later than normal depending on which way the time difference is. You can then take the next dose close to your usual time, in the new time zone. Within 48 hours you should have adapted to the new time zone. Remember to do this on the way back too!

Sun protection

If you have a transplant, you are three times more likely than other people to develop skin cancer (see page 115). This is because of the immunosuppressant drugs you need to take. However, there are precautions you can take which will reduce your risk. You should stay indoors, or at least in the shade, between 10 am and 2 pm, when the sun's UV rays are at their strongest. When you do go out, always use a strong sunblock with an SPF (sun protection factor) of at least 25. You should also protect your skin by wearing suitable clothing. Long-sleeved shirts with collars, and hats are a good idea. Be aware that many summer-weight fabrics don't give enough protection and fibres like cotton offer even less protection when wet.

It is a good idea to wear sunglasses that block 99–100 % of UV radiation. Check the label when you buy them.

You should avoid using sun beds to develop a tan before you go away.

Examine your skin regularly. If you find any unusual blemishes or moles, especially one that changes in size, shape or colour, see your doctor.

Avoiding infections

Transplant immunosuppressant drugs reduce your ability to fight infections. Simple precautions include the following:

- Avoid contact with people who have a cold, 'flu, or any infectious diseases such as chicken pox. (It's not possible or practical to avoid contact with people who have minor infections.)

- Don't drink local water in poorly developed countries. Boil the water or buy bottled water.

- Again, in poorly developed countries, avoid salads unless you have washed them yourself, and avoid ice cubes unless you have made them yourself from bottled water.

- Avoid ice cream from street vendors.

- Avoid travelling to countries where the risk of catching an infection is high. British Airways Clinics can advise you. Make sure you know in advance where the nearest transplant unit is (don't rely on any local doctor). If you are going to be more than 24–36 hours away from anywhere, maybe think twice about where you are going.

Be prepared

It is worth taking a basic first aid kit, including an emergency supply of plasters, bandages, antiseptic cream, painkillers, syringes/needles, insect repellent, insect bite ointment and anti-diarrhoea tablets.

It is safest to divide your supply of tablets. Keep half with you in your hand luggage, and pack the other half in the luggage you check in, or give it to a companion to carry.

You will need a letter from your doctor stating that the drugs you are carrying are prescription drugs. It is a good idea to carry a letter stating you are a transplant patient and are fit to travel. This is particularly helpful in some countries, and with some insurance companies.

It is useful to carry a written list of all the details of your medications, including the prescription names (as written on the label), the dosages, and how often you take them – so that if your supply is lost, you can advise doctors accordingly.

It is also worth taking contact details, email addresses and phone numbers for your kidney unit, along with your consultant's name – in case someone needs to call to check on your drugs or medical history if anything were to go wrong. The unexpected can happen and so can accidents. Ensuring you have contact information is one simple way of making life safer and easier in the event of problems.

If you need to take medication that must be kept cool, pack it in a small picnic cool bag or a jiffy bag with ice packs, or use a wide-necked thermos flask which has been chilled. Make sure you allow time for transfers and delays when calculating the length of your journey.

On your return trip, remember to declare to customs any drugs you were given or prescribed. Remember to check whether any additional security measures are in place, for example stringent restrictions on hand luggage (as was the case at UK airports in the summer of 2006).

If you are travelling within the European Union, make sure you have a European Health Insurance Card (EHIC). You can pick up an application form from your local post office or apply online at www.ehic.org.uk/Internet/home.dh. It is also advisable to have additional travel insurance, particularly if you are travelling outside the European Union. The NKF Helpline (see Appendix 2) can give you more advice about insurance.

EATING AND DRINKING

If you have been on dialysis, what you eat and how much you can drink may have been severely restricted for quite a long time. You will have had to avoid foods containing certain substances such as sodium and potassium, and the amount of water and other fluids will have been restricted.

ENJOYING YOUR FREEDOM
WHILE KEEPING YOUR KIDNEY HEALTHY

One of the many good things about having a transplant is that it releases you from the drudgery of the dietary and fluid restrictions of dialysis. When your transplant is working well, you may well feel like going out and having bags of crisps and chocolates every day. That is fine for a few days. In the long term, however, it is not a good thing. Remember if you are on steroids, your appetite will always be good, perhaps too good. So you will have to be very controlled if you are to avoid putting on weight and becoming obese. Like everything else in life, you need to find a balance between enjoying the dietary freedom of a transplant but not eat so much that your weight makes you ill. Maybe eat out about once a week, then do not go too mad. Obesity can cause diabetes and high blood pressure, either of which can contribute to early failure of your kidney. You may not feel like eating if you are back on dialysis.

ASHOK: ENJOYING FOOD AGAIN

Ashok was 53 when, after five years of dialysis, he finally received a transplant. The operation went well and he was thrilled to discover how much better he felt.

Before he became ill, Ashok loved his food. Sita, his wife, is a splendid cook and although she tried hard to prepare meals that Ashok could eat, he badly missed her wonderful curries, so rich in potassium and salt. What was worse, he found that his sense of taste altered while he was on dialysis, so he could not enjoy the sweetmeats that were served at every family celebration. To Ashok's delight, he discovered that his tastebuds returned to normal after his operation – and so did Sita's cooking. But after some months, his kidney doctor warned him that he was putting on too much weight. In addition, several members of Ashok's extended family have Type 2 diabetes and although he does not have it himself yet, he is thought to be at very high risk of developing it.

Ashok was referred to a renal dietitian who spent some time talking with him and Sita about their lifestyle and food preferences. She drew up a diet plan for Ashok, and so far (it has been five months now) this seems to be working well. Ashok is sure that part of the reason he is able to follow the plan is that it takes into account what sort of food he enjoys, and gives him room for the occasional treat.

KEEPING FIT

Many people find they have much more energy once they have recovered from transplant surgery. This is particularly likely to be the case if they have been on dialysis for some years. So it is important to enjoy this new-found sense of well-being and do whatever you can to maintain it for as long as possible.

Everyone, whatever their age or health status, is likely to benefit from some sort of regular, moderate exercise. Programmes have been devised even for people who are chair-bound. But now you are free from dialysis the chances are you can do something rather more interesting than that.

A note of caution however: if you have been inactive for a long time (which may well be the case if you have been on dialysis) you might need to ease into a routine slowly and carefully. It would be a good idea to start by talking to your doctor as he or she will tell you if there are any reasons why you need to be extra careful, or any movements or types of sport you should avoid. Generally speaking, people with a kidney transplant are advised to avoid contact sports such as judo as they might be at risk of damaging the new kidney. They might also be advised to avoid anything that causes the blood pressure to rise too sharply.

Most people will not be tempted to train for a marathon, they just want to find a way to keep their heart and limbs in good working order, preferably by doing something they enjoy. Some people enjoy salsa dancing; others may prefer swimming or running. Regular, brisk walking has many advantages and is easy to build into your daily routine. Don't forget that digging, pushing a lawn mower, and pulling up weeds can all be forms of exercise – and have the advantage of being carried out in the open air. A physiotherapist will talk through with you ways of building exercise into your daily life so that you find it enjoyable and not disruptive. If you can find ways of keeping fit that are fun as well, and that do not eat into the time you set aside for other activities, you are much more likely to stick with them and see real benefits.

KEY FACTS

1. After a transplant you are likely to feel much better in yourself as well, and have more energy to enjoy life.

2. Taking your medication every day and keeping fit are very important.

3. Many of the restrictions of dialysis (such as diet and the amount of liquid you can drink) are no longer necessary.

4. Work and holidays become much easier to manage.

5. Travelling abroad needs advance planning to reduce the risks of infection.

6. Transplant patients should seek specialist advice before having any vaccination.

12
Relationships, sex and having children

This chapter looks at the changes having a transplant might make to your intimate relationships, and how a successful transplant might affect your plans for having a family.

Most people find that they feel much fitter after they have had a kidney transplant. This usually means that they have more energy and a better sex drive than before the operation. The high level of waste that has been present in the body before a transplant goes down to more normal levels and the body can work much better. However, a good sex life is not guaranteed. There may have been serious problems on dialysis that cannot be reversed. Diabetes, stress, or side effects of drugs can affect sex drive. In addition, many people feel quite depressed for a while after a major operation (see pages 98–100) and this can affect your sex drive too. You may find your emotions are quite complicated if you have received a kidney for transplant from your partner, and don't forget that a healthy person who has had an operation to remove a kidney will find they too feel more tired than usual for some weeks afterwards.

The doctors and nurses in the transplant clinic will be able to advise on ways in which sex life may be improved after a transplant. Don't be embarrassed to ask them for advice – they have worked with very many patients and are committed to helping restore your quality of life.

Although immediately after a transplant, sex would probably not damage the kidney, it is sensible to refrain from sex for about four weeks. Anyway, you may not feel like it until you have recovered a bit from the operation.

DRUGS TO HELP WITH ERECTIONS

Although sex drive returns for many patients, others may still have problems. This can be a real problem and one that can be difficult to talk about. Many men on dialysis find both their libido and their ability to have an erection is greatly improved by taking an erythropoiesis-stimulating agent (ESA or EPO), as anaemia is a major cause of tiredness and erection difficulties. Getting a transplant means that many people can come off their ESA treatment, but unfortunately this does not apply to everyone. Perhaps as many as 25% find they need to keep on with ESA, for a few weeks at least.

If erection problems are not caused by anaemia, however, other help is available. The tablet Viagra (sildenafil) can be prescribed to men after a transplant. Many have found it has helped them get or maintain an erection. However, it may not be safe for some patients with heart problems. There are other similar drugs available now, such as cialis, but again these will not be suitable for everyone. If your doctor thinks that these medicines are not safe for you, there are other treatments available that help men get erections. These treatments may involve injections into the penis, or squirting a drug into the opening at the end of the penis. This latter technique is called MUSE (medicated urethral system for erections).

A specialist on impotence (otherwise known as an erectile dysfunction or ED specialist) can advise you. The specialist will also check that ED is not caused by another reason entirely, as many of these (such as testosterone deficiency) are reasonably straightforward to treat.

CONTRACEPTION

The combined Pill is safe for most women to take after a transplant, particularly a tablet that is low in oestrogen. However it is best avoided in those who have high blood pressure or blood clotting problems. Some women, such as those who are older, for whom the combined Pill is not suitable, may find the progesterone-only Pill a good alternative. If you want to use another method of contraception, such as the coil (intra-uterine device), diaphragm or condoms, do talk to your doctor first to make sure that they are suitable for you in your particular circumstances.

If you do not have a long-term partner, then be sure to practise 'safe sex'. Condoms are known to reduce your likelihood of getting AIDS and other sexually transmitted diseases such as gonorrhoea. Don't forget that taking immunosuppressant medication will make you more vulnerable to infections of every kind.

PLANNING A PREGNANCY

Most people find that, while their fertility may be reduced when they are on dialysis, it usually returns to normal levels after a transplant. This is true for men as well as for women, but it is perhaps particularly relevant for women as it is rare to have a successful pregnancy while on dialysis.

Most women under about 50 find their periods return to a normal pattern as the levels of toxins in the body go down, allowing the balance of hormones to be restored. Oestradiol is one of the hormones that controls women's periods, and this is usually restored to normal levels after a transplant. This results in ovulation (egg production in the ovaries) starting up again, and a restoration of fertility. Some women have irregular or very frequent periods until things 'settle down', which may take six months or more. Others may be fertile very soon after a transplant, so all women should take precautions.

Women who have been on dialysis for a time, then have a transplant, may find that they develop breast lumps. There can be several of these, and a doctor should always check them. However, they are much more likely to be benign than cancerous.

If you are a woman who has just had a transplant and wants to start a family (or have another child), your doctor is likely to discourage you from getting pregnant for at least a year after your operation. Pregnancy can cause problems with the levels of immunosuppressant drugs in your body, as well as making your blood pressure go up. So you will be doing your body a favour if you give the new kidney a chance to get well 'settled in' before you try to get pregnant.

During your pregnancy, you are likely to find yourself being cared for jointly by both the kidney transplant team and the maternity team. They will work together with your GP and midwife throughout your pregnancy. It is very important that your kidney function and your blood pressure are monitored on a regular basis throughout your pregnancy.

Table 12.1 shows the percentage chance of problems occurring for mothers who have a transplant in one research study, depending on the level of creatinine in the blood.

There is also a risk that your transplant kidney may be damaged during pregnancy, although it is rare for the pregnancy to cause the transplant to fail. The level of your blood creatinine level at the time you get pregnant is really important. If it is less than 100 mmol/L, there will be almost no risk of damaging the transplant kidney. However, if your blood creatinine level is between 100 and 130 mmol/L during the pregnancy, there is a 15%

Table 12.1 Risk of pregnancy-related problems for kidney transplant patients

	Creatinine less than 120 mmol/L	Creatinine of more than 120 mmol/L
Chance of problems during pregnancy	30%	82%
Chance of a successful pregnancy	97%	75%
Chance of the mother having long-term problems	7%	27%

GLENDA: RUNNING OUT OF TIME?

Glenda is 37 years old and wants to have a baby. She feels she is running out of time to get pregnant. Her husband Steve would like a baby but not if it means Glenda risking her health. She has had Type 1 diabetes (requiring insulin) since the age of 14. She has, by and large, looked after herself. She has a creatinine of 250 μmol/L (which means she is about three years away from needing dialysis).

Glenda's doctor advised her not to start trying for a baby, as it would be very unlikely to survive. He said it would be safer to start dialysis about a year earlier than planned. She didn't believe her doctor and did get pregnant. Sadly she had a miscarriage. To make it worse, her blood pressure went through the roof, and she needed to start dialysis within days of the miscarriage. Her doctor turned out to have been right.

Fortunately, after a period of temporary haemodialysis, Glenda settled down well on to APD. She was told that if she was transplanted, her fertility would return though it would be a good idea to wait a year after the transplant. She had a kidney-pancreas transplant six months later, and both kidney and pancreas worked well. So she came off dialysis, her diabetes was 'cured', and she was able to stop taking insulin. After a year, she did become pregnant and gave birth to a lovely boy called Joshua. In a way she was glad she had the miscarriage and rapid passage to dialysis, as she would never have had the transplant, and so never had Joshua. If this hadn't happened her kidneys could have deteriorated slowly until she was 40, by which time her fertility could have been markedly reduced.

chance that your transplant will fail within eight years. If your creatinine level is more than 130 mmol/L when you become pregnant, however, your kidney has a one in three chance of failing within three years. In addition, your blood pressure level is likely to go up (this happens in many pregnant women, not just those who have had transplants). In addition, the levels of ciclosporin and other drugs in your blood will fall (because of the increased fluid volume in your body), meaning the dose taken has to be increased. A few women find the effectiveness of their transplanted kidney will be permanently reduced after pregnancy.

A common worry is that the drugs given to prevent rejection and all the other problems of transplantation will cause damage to the baby. Surprisingly, this is not a major problem, although research does suggest that women with a kidney transplant may be slightly more likely than other women to have a miscarriage early on in the pregnancy. When the pregnancy does progress, however, the baby will be at no greater risk of abnormalities than babies born to healthy women. The blood pressure often rises quite high at about 34 weeks of pregnancy, and the situation can become sufficiently serious for the baby to need to be delivered a little prematurely. As long as this is anticipated, there are unlikely to be serious problems as a result. This is one of the reasons transplant units usually suggest that the birth takes place in the same hospital as the transplant unit, where staff will have more experience of pregnant women with transplants.

Breastfeeding may not be possible after delivery, depending on the drugs being taken for the transplant. Ciclosporin comes through the body into breast milk so, if the mother is taking this drug, the baby will have to be bottle-fed.

KEY FACTS

1 Fertility and sex drive can improve after a transplant.

2 For a man, a successful transplant may improve erectile dysfunction. If it doesn't, sildenafil (Viagra) may help.

3 A woman can get pregnant very soon after a transplant, so take precautions.

4 Women who have had a transplant are advised not to get pregnant for a year after the transplant operation.

5 There are risks to both mother and baby – although, if the kidney is working well, the risks are less.

13
Transplant failure

In this chapter we explain what can be done to postpone the eventual failure of your transplant. We talk about the causes of transplant kidney failure, give advice on how to cope and discuss the options available to you afterwards.

A kidney transplant does not last forever. The average life span of a transplanted kidney is 10 years for a deceased donor transplant, and about 15 years for one from a living donor. So younger patients may need two or more transplants in their lives. If a transplant fails, you can restart dialysis, and you may be able to go back on the transplant waiting list.

SUCCESS RATE FOR SECOND TRANSPLANTS

The success rate for second transplants is almost as good as for first transplants, once a suitable kidney has been found. If a second transplant fails, then a third and even fourth transplant can sometimes be performed.

CAUSES OF TRANSPLANT FAILURE

The most common cause for transplant failure is rejection. 'Rejection' means that the patient's body recognises that the transplanted kidney is not 'its own' and tries to 'reject' it from the body. Even when patients and transplant kidneys are apparently 'well-matched' (in terms of blood group and tissue type, see Chapter 2), some degree of rejection is common. The severity of rejection varies from patient to patient. Rejection may be either acute (see pages 90–93) or chronic (see page 105). Rejection can occur if the dose of the anti-rejection drugs is wrong or if the patient doesn't take their immunosuppressant drugs properly.

Other causes of transplant failure are:

- Infection;

- Blood clots that stop or reduce the blood supply to the new kidney;

- A return of the disease that caused kidney failure in the first place.

Return of the original disease is rare as there are only a few diseases that will return in a transplanted kidney. What is more, it is likely to be many years before the disease does significant damage to the new kidney. If it should happen, however, there is a chance that the same thing could happen in a second transplant. Should you be unlucky enough to find yourself in this situation, your doctor will take it extremely seriously. He or she will discuss fully with you the chances of this happening with a second transplant, the rate at which problems might develop, and what can be done about the situation. Many people can be transplanted a second time, but the risks should be assessed on an individual basis.

HOW DOES REJECTION CAUSE TRANSPLANT FAILURE?

Acute rejection can occur during the first three months after the transplant and cause the transplant to fail rapidly, over a period of a few days. Or it can damage a kidney so badly that it fails over a few weeks or months after the transplant. Acute rejection is less common after the first few months, but can occur, particularly if someone stops taking their medication, or has another illness that stops the medication being absorbed into the body.

However, these days very few transplants fail from acute rejection. It is more common for transplants to fail from chronic rejection, or 'chronic allograft nephropathy'. This is a slow process, taking months or years to cause transplant failure. A very low level of rejection in the kidney is followed by damage and scarring that is caused by several other factors, such as high blood pressure or excessive levels of immunosuppressant drugs that are toxic to the kidney (see Chapter 8).

If you know your transplant is starting to fail and you are beginning to feel the symptoms of kidney failure again, you should talk to your doctor. You can suggest that you start planning to re-start dialysis and go back onto the transplant list. You could also talk about the possibility of having a living donor transplant, if you have a suitable donor. Try not to feel intimidated by the doctors. You will know how you feel and good planning can help prevent problems.

Sometimes people develop heart disease or other medical problems after they have had a transplant. If these problems are serious, they may make having a second transplant dangerous. When your transplant starts to fail, you will have tests to make sure you are fit enough for a second transplant. These will be very similar to the fitness tests carried out before you had your first transplant.

ARE ALL PATIENTS WHO HAVE A FAILED TRANSPLANT ENTITLED TO ANOTHER?

If someone has had a transplant that failed because they did not take their tablets, or did not turn up regularly for clinic appointments, some doctors may fear that the person will not 'look after' their new transplant. Many doctors and nurses feel it would be a waste of a scarce resource to put them on the transplant list and give them a kidney that someone else might take much better care of. Doctors therefore act as 'gatekeepers' and may stop people going on the transplant list, whatever the patient's wishes.

Some people who have lost a transplant because they have not taken tablets or attended clinics do eventually go back onto the transplant list, or receive a living donor kidney. Before this can happen, there needs to be an understanding that the person's ability to cope with stress has improved, or at least that they can cope better with the problems that led to the initial cause of transplant failure. Usually several people on the transplant team will make an assessment, and if someone has been seeing a psychologist or another professional providing support, their involvement will be helpful. If someone is not attending all their dialysis sessions or clinic appointments, or taking their prescribed medication, the transplant team will be reluctant to re-transplant someone, even if they want another kidney and say they will take their medication in the future.

WAITING FOR A KIDNEY AFTER TRANSPLANT FAILURE

There can be a long wait for another kidney after one has failed. The body has a powerful memory for the tissue types in the first transplant. This means that the immune system is pre-programmed to reject a new kidney almost as soon as it is placed the body. This usually means that patients have to wait longer for a well-matched kidney the second time around.

It is even more difficult for some patients to get a second transplant because the failed kidney causes the body to produce antibodies. These antibodies are programmed to attack the tissue types of the original kidney. However they can also react to other similar tissue types. This may mean that someone has antibodies that will react with any new kidneys, even if the tissue type match is nearly perfect. The antibodies will cause a positive cross-match test (see page 13) and make transplantation very difficult. Doctors have tried to find ways of removing these antibodies, but the techniques are still experimental; they have side effects and are not always successful.

COPING WITH A FAILED TRANSPLANT

The failure of a kidney transplant can have a massive impact on a person's life – not just on their physical condition. A person's psychological and emotional well-being can also have an effect on their physical well-being.

The way people behave can have a direct effect on their physical condition. If someone is told that their transplant kidney is starting to fail, they may feel low and depressed and become less careful about taking their medication. This will only add to the problem.

If their failing kidney was from a living donor, the relationship can suffer unless people are able to be open, honest and non-judgemental.

BERNARD: COPING WITH FAILURE FOR SOMEONE ELSE

Bernard is 62. Seven years ago he had a kidney transplant after being offered a kidney by his brother Kevin, who is five years younger. Now the kidney is beginning to fail and Bernard has been told he is likely to need to go back on dialysis in about six months.

Bernard has read that the average lifespan of a living donor kidney transplant is 15 years. He wonders why his kidney is giving up early – has he done something wrong? He hasn't said anything to Kevin yet. He is worried that his brother will demand to know why Bernard couldn't look after the kidney properly.

If Bernard did feel able to discuss the issue with Kevin, he would find his brother much more sympathetic than he fears. Kevin has always looked up to his 'big' brother and feels that he has been really brave all through his illness. He is glad to have given Bernard some dialysis-free years, but would be sorry that 'his' kidney didn't keep going for his brother for longer.

Unfortunately, fears about how Kevin will react have become the focus for Bernard's distress and worry about having to go back on dialysis. He is grieving for the failing kidney and the loss of control over his life that losing it will bring, but he cannot face telling his brother. Kevin hasn't been able to speak to his brother for three months as Bernard won't answer the phone himself anymore, and doesn't return calls. Kevin misses their friendship and wonders what he has done wrong.

STRESS FOR KIDNEY TRANSPLANT PATIENTS

Any long-term illness or surgical operation can be extremely stressful. In fact any change – even a pleasant change like getting married – is stressful. Similarly, a 'good' thing like a having a transplant can be stressful. When changes are 'negative', for example if the transplant fails, stress will be greatly increased.

Some of the stresses that commonly affect people with a failed kidney transplant are:

- Taking in strange information, to enable them to understand a complex medical subject;

- Learning about themselves and the ways they cope with things;

- Needing to ask for support to manage the transplant failure;

- Worrying about the future.

Other members of the family also have to make adjustments. Kidney transplant failure has an impact on their lives too. The normal pattern of life is disrupted and relationships have to be redefined. This may be particularly difficult if the patient received the first kidney from a loved one. If the person has to go back on dialysis, particularly if they have never had dialysis before, the impact on the family can be huge.

Initial reactions

Being told that your kidney transplant is failing can be devastating. Many people have waited a long time to have a transplant and be free from the restrictions of dialysis. Being told that it is failing can sometimes be as – or even more – difficult to cope with as the original diagnosis of kidney failure. Patients can go through the following emotions:

1. **Shock** – At first, patients (and sometimes also family members and friends) go into a state of shock, feeling stunned, bewildered or strangely detached – as though they are observing life rather than being part of it. This shock can last a short while or may continue for weeks.

2. **Grief** – Then people begin to react to the news, often with feelings of loss, sadness, helplessness and despair. They may feel overwhelmed by reality, and find it difficult to think clearly or plan effectively.

❸ **Denial** – One very common reaction to a failing transplant is to deny the diagnosis or its implications.

❹ **Acceptance** – Gradually, people come to accept reality a little at a time, and begin to make progress towards adapting successfully to the prospect of life back on dialysis.

Longer-term problems

Some people can experience longer-term psychological problems when their transplant fails. Some of these are described below.

Awareness of early death

People with kidney failure know that without treatment they would die. Having a transplant makes patients feel more 'normal' and some of the anxiety associated with living on dialysis can go away. However, when the transplant fails, fears of dying are likely to return. People who live with this sort of knowledge have a very different perspective on life and its priorities.

Dependency and loss of self-confidence

Kidney patients are very dependent on many people. They are dependent on hospital doctors and nurses, and on their partners, relatives and friends. People with kidney failure have to deal with the fact that their life depends on a machine or on a regular supply of PD bags. Even people who have had a transplant can feel dependent on someone else's kidney. This necessary dependency can undermine a person's ability to cope with both kidney and non-kidney issues. They may wonder if they are 'doing it right', for example. Or they may worry about becoming dependent on someone of whom they are used to 'taking care'. Often, patients who have had a transplant can regain some of their independence; however, when the kidney fails, the problems recur.

If issues relating to dependency and self-confidence are not dealt with, they may cause conflict between kidney patients and hospital staff or carers.

Sense of loss

The loss of the tranplant kidney is a substantial loss, and needs to be acknowledged as such. People who have a failed transplant may feel responsibility or guilt for the kidney's failure. They may worry that they should have done something different to prevent it from failing.

Depression

Most people get depressed at some stage in their lives. Periods of depression may be useful, in that they enable people to withdraw from the world for a while, and resolve certain issues. People with kidney failure are no exception. There are times when they feel low, and to do anything at all requires a huge effort; times when they should allow themselves to feel sorry about themselves; and times to cry. When a transplant fails, it is important to understand that depression is a 'normal' emotion.

FACTORS AFFECTING THE ABILITY TO COPE

Some people cope more easily than others with the psychological and emotional aspects of a failed kidney transplant. A person's ability to cope with transplant failure is influenced by a range of factors.

Age

The age at which a person experiences a failed kidney transplant is likely to influence the way they will cope:

- Children may not understand the long-term implications of the condition.

- Adolescents need to be liked and accepted by their peers. Having a transplant makes them appear more normal, and they may find going onto dialysis particularly difficult to cope with.

- Young adults may feel they no longer have the chance to develop their lives in the direction they planned – to get married, to have children or to enter a particular career. Such feelings may cause anger and resentment.

- Middle-aged patients may have problems adjusting to the disruption of an established lifestyle.

- Older patients may resent not being able to enjoy their retirement, or look after their grandchildren.

Personality

Aspects of a patient's personality can affect their ability to cope with the failure of a kidney transplant:

- People who cope well with long-term health problems tend to have hardy or resilient personalities which allow them to see good in difficult situations.

- They are able to balance hope against despair and to find purpose in life whatever happens. They maintain their self-esteem and resist feeling helpless and hopeless.

Social and cultural factors
A person's ability to cope with illness is also affected by their background:

- People from different social, cultural and religious backgrounds will have different ways of dealing with situations. Problems may arise if doctors and nurses fail to take this into account.

- People's beliefs about health come from a number of sources, including the media, advertising, other patients' experiences and their friends. These beliefs may be incorrect or only half true. This is one of the reasons why we have written this book.

Support
The amount and quality of support available to patients further influences how well they cope with the failure of their transplant:

- People who live alone, away from their family and with few friends, tend to adjust poorly to long-term diseases. Other forms of support are particularly important for people in this position.

- The immediate family is the main source of psychological support for many people. But for others, this role is taken by one or more close friends. Such support is usually a big help to the patient. However, it is also true that relatives and friends sometimes undermine effective coping by providing bad examples or poor advice.

- Hospitals do not always provide patients with the support they need when their transplant fails. Hospitals can be dull places for patients, and further depress their mood. Unfortunately, at present, very few kidney units include a clinical psychologist on the staff. However, there is a general recognition of the need to provide patients with psychological support, and some nurses have had special training in counselling.

- Many support groups have been set up by, and for, people with kidney failure. These groups can provide emotional and sometimes financial support, as well as information (see Appendix 2).

KEY FACTS

❶ A kidney transplant will not last a lifetime.

❷ When the kidney transplant fails, dialysis or another transplant will be needed.

❸ The success rate of a second transplant is as good as for the first one.

❹ The most common cause of transplant failure is chronic rejection.

❺ There are things you can do to slow down the failure of the kidney, such as keeping your blood pressure low.

❻ Coping with a failed transplant can be difficult.

14
Research and future developments

In this chapter we look at the history of transplantation and discuss the possible future of kidney transplants.

HISTORY OF TRANSPLANTATION – A TIME OF RAPID CHANGE

Transplantation has changed rapidly in the last 50 years. The first successful human kidney transplant was from a living donor. It was performed on 23 December 1954 by Dr Joseph Murray and his team at the Peter Bent Brigham Hospital, Boston, USA. A kidney was removed from one man and transplanted into his genetically identical twin brother. The transplant was performed between identical twins because it was known that rejection would cause the failure of a transplant between people who were not genetically identical. In 1954 there were no drugs to prevent rejection occurring.

The first drug that was used to prevent rejection was azathioprine in 1963. Azathioprine is still used in some transplants performed in the 21st century. However, in the early days of transplantation, 3 out of 10 transplants failed in the first year – even when azathioprine was used. Despite these poor success rates, transplantion was soon being performed in many countries throughout the world.

A drug called ciclosporin was developed in the early 1980s and was seen as revolutionary in the prevention of transplant rejection. Almost immediately, it was succesful in further reducing the early failure rate of transplants to 2 out of 10. Since the late 1990s, the early failure rate of transplants has dropped again to about 1 in 10. This is partly because of new drugs that have become available, but it is also due to the use of new and better anaesthetics used during the transplant operation itself, as well as to better ways of diagnosing and treating infection.

In the UK, in the late 1990s, with deceased donor kidneys becoming less available, living donor transplantation has become much more common. Antibody incompatible (and exchange) transplantation (see page 59), are examples of progress in the 21st century. Even though the results are no better than 'ordinary transplants', giving a chance to patients who would never normally get a kidney is a major advance.

WHAT IS RESEARCH AND HOW DOES IT APPLY TO ME?

If you have a kidney transplant, you are benefitting from research performed over the last 50 years. All transplant units carry out research to try to keep on improving the results of kidney transplantation. Many people who have a kidney transplant will be asked to take part in some research. It is important to understand your options if you are asked to take part in any reseach project.

Medical research projects are all reviewed by an independent Ethics Committee. The doctors who want to do the research have to describe in detail exactly what procedures are involved in the study, and how many people will be asked to take part. The written information that people see when they are asked to take part is reviewed to make sure it is accurate and can be understood. Every patient taking part in a research study has to be fully informed, and has to agree to take part. There are some exceptions to this, for example the Ethics Committee may agree that some research can be performed without individual consent on blood samples left over after normal tests have been performed. In a case like this, no effect on the individuals themselves is possible, as the samples have already left the body.

Every patient has the right to refuse to take part in a research study, or to withdraw from it at any time without giving a reason. Doctors may be disappointed if someone doesn't agree to take part in some research, but they are not allowed to let this affect the patient's treatment in any way. So no one should feel under any pressure to take part in a research study, and must have as long as possible to think about whether to take part. Do not be pressurised into making an immediate decision.

Broadly speaking, there are two types of research:

1. Research into a new treatment, and

2. Research into the general effects of a transplant. This is done simply by taking extra blood samples, or performing some sort of test, but the patients' treatment is left alone.

TAKING PART IN A RESEARCH STUDY: WHAT DO YOU NEED TO KNOW?

You are under no obligation to take part in research, although it is great if you do, as research helps to improve treatments for future patients. It is because other patients have done so before you, that a transplant is possible for you today. You should be sure the nurse or doctor running the study answers the following questions:

- What is the background to the study, and why is it being done?
- What will you have to do?
- How long will the study last?
- What are the potential side effects of the study?
- How does being in the research differ from normal care?
- Will information from the study be kept confidential?
- Will information be used to write articles for the medical press, and could this information get into the national press?
- Will any side effects from the drugs in the trials be reported to the Committee for the Safety of Medicines?
- Can you get compensation for any expenses you may have? For example, taxi fares or petrol and parking for extra trips to the hospital required by the study?
- Has the study been approved by the local Research Ethics Committee, or the Multicentre Research Ethics Committee (for a national study)?
- If the trial is being sponsored by a drug company, have they signed up to compensation guidelines and do they have insurance against any problems that might occur?
- Have you been told whether the company sponsoring the study will have access to your medical records to verify results and examinations?
- Will your future treatment be affected by whether or not you take part in the study?

After consenting to take part in the study, you will be seen frequently by members of staff from the research team (usually nurses) for the duration of the study. You should be given clear instructions as to whom, exactly, you should contact if you have any questions or concerns during the period of the study. Some drug trials will include a 24-hour helpline.

If you are asked to take part in a research study involving medications, you should be told very clearly whether the drug you are being offered is completely new, or whether the study is looking at combinations of drugs that have already been used separately. The side effects of the drugs should be explained clearly to you, and you should be given written information about them to read and take away with you.

Most drug studies compare two or three different types of drug treatment. To make a valid comparison of the treatments, neither you nor your doctor can decide which of the treatment options you will be getting. The drugs are allocated to each patient according to a secret code. This is called 'randomisation', and is an important part of well-managed drug trials. It is essential that you are told whether your treatment will be randomised when you are asked to take part in a study. But once you have agreed to take part and signed all the forms, you will not know which of the treatment options is the one you are getting. When the trial is over you can ask your doctors to find out.

JENNIFER: TAKING PART IN A DRUG TRIAL

Jennifer is 42, and had a transplant eight months ago. The new kidney is working well.

On visiting the clinic, Jennifer is asked to take part in a trial of a new immunosuppressant treatment. It is explained to her that this will be a 'double blind randomised controlled trial'. So she will not know whether her existing treatment regime is continuing (albeit with different-coloured tablets), or whether she will be on a new mix of drugs including one which is not generally available. Her doctor will not know either – that is what 'double-blind' means. She is given written information about the trial and asked to go away and think more about it.

Jennifer discusses the idea with Nigel, her partner. They decide that as she has been lucky enough to get a transplant after waiting just nine months, she would like to 'give something back', so she agrees to participate.

Jennifer starts on the 'new' tablet regime, not knowing whether the drugs she is taking have changed. Unfortunately, after several weeks, she develops an infection with stomach pain and nausea that is quite severe. Not knowing whether this is because her treatment has changed, she becomes worried and asks whether she can leave the trial and return to her original treatment. It was explained to her before the trial started that she would have a right to do this and her future treatment would in no way be affected by such a decision.

Six months on, Jennifer worries that she made a mistake. She now suspects she may have been on exactly the same medication all along and that the infection was due to unrelated causes.

She tells Pam, her transplant nurse, that she feels really guilty about letting the team down. Pam reassures her that pulling out of the trial when she was worried and unwell was entirely appropriate. The most important thing is for her to look after her health and the new kidney.

In the second type of research, extra blood tests will be taken, or some other kind of investigation will be performed. The results of the test are compared with the what happens to you (and to your kidney) in the longer term – for example, if you have an episode of rejection. As this type of study does not involve taking any new or experimental drugs, many people find it is not difficult to agree to take part. However, it is worth checking in advance whether a research study of this type involves extra clinic visits over and above the routine requirements.

POSSIBLE FUTURE DEVELOPMENTS

Drug treatments

Although many of the drugs that are used today have been prescribed in kidney transplantation for years, this does not mean that the best ways to use them are fully understood. There are also new drugs coming out, especially ones that are given by injection around the time of the transplant to reduce early rejection rates.

A few examples of newer drugs or areas of interest are given below, but this list is not exhaustive, and some of these questions may be answered in the near future.

❶ **Drugs that kill white blood cells** There is interest in drugs that kill many of the white blood cells in the body. Since the white blood cells cause rejection, the drug may reduce early rejection rates. The drugs currently used tend to reduce the activity of white blood cells, rather than removing them completely. It is hoped that the use of more potent drugs soon after the transplant may allow lower doses of drugs to be given in the longer term, giving better results. One drug of this type is alemtuzumab (also called Campath), and is given by injection around the time of the transplant.

❷ **Drugs that kill selected types of white blood cells** There is a lot of interest in a type of drug that kills just one type of white blood cell, called 'B cells'. These are involved in the rejection process, and also develop into cells that produce antibodies that can be damaging to the transplant. Rituximab is the name of the drug that is currently most used for this purpose. It is given by injection, and is being used in a number of studies.

❸ **Reducing long-term side effects** Trials are in progress to see if the long term side effects of drugs can be reduced by switching between different drugs, or using new drugs. Because ciclosporin and tacrolimus can be toxic (poisonous) to the kidney, there are trials which try and stop them altogether, or to reduce their dosage markedly. Another long-term side effect of immunosuppressant drugs is cancer, especially skin cancers. Trials are in progress to see whether switching to the immunosuppressant drug sirolimus reduces the risk of skin cancers. As well as having an immuno-suppressant action, sirolimus has an anti-cancer action, so it may be able to provide a dual effect.

❹ **Long-term treatment using injections** This research is at an early stage but is examining the possibility that long-term immunosuppression would be achieved by giving drugs through a drip one day a month, and reducing or stopping the daily tablets.

NEW THERAPIES

Although the results of transplantation have improved markedly in the last 10 years, it would be better if successful transplantation did not rely on the long-term use of immunosuppressant drugs, and a great deal of work is being performed to see if newer approaches could eliminate the use of these drugs. This would be the 'Holy Grail' of transplantation, but is currently not possible.

Xenotransplantation

The term 'xenotransplantation' refers to the possibility of using organs (such as kidneys) taken from animals, especially pigs, for transplantation into humans. A certain amount of research has been done in this area, but the problems are currently considered to be too great. One major concern is the risk of passing on animal viruses to humans.

Stem cell 'kidneys'

Research is also being carried out to see if kidneys can be grown or repaired using stem cells. These are very simple cells (the microscopic building blocks of nature) taken from an adult (or human fetus) that can be made to develop into more mature, kidney-like, cells.

Although this research has received considerable publicity, and might change the face of kidney failure in years to come, it is unlikely to help people with kidney failure in the near future.

KEY FACTS

1. The first kidney transplant was performed in 1954. There have been major advances in the treatment since then.

2. Advances in kidney transplants would not be possible without research.

3. Taking part in a research study makes you part of the history of transplantation.

4. There are two main types of kidney transplant research:

   (a) Research into new drugs to prevent rejection;

   (b) Research into the general effects of a transplant.

5. Participating in research is entirely voluntary.

6. Make sure you fully understand the study before agreeing to take part in any research.

7. New treatments are being developed all the time, but major changes to transplantation are unlikely in the near future.

Glossary

This glossary provides brief explanations of the various technical words and abbreviations used in this book. Words printed in *italic* type have their own glossary entry.

Abdomen The lower part of the trunk, below the chest. Commonly called the tummy or belly.

Acute A word meaning short term and of rapid onset, usually requiring a rapid response.

Acute rejection Rejection that develops acutely, and requires immediate action. Usually diagnosed with a biopsy, and treated with high dose steroids or, if resistant, with *ATG* or *OKT3*.

AIT Abbreviation for *antibody incompatible transplantation*.

Alemtuzumab A new drug, also known as *Campath*, currently being tested in research trials. It could be an alternative to *basiliximab* or *daclizumab*.

ALG Abbreviation for anti-lymphocyte globulin, a strong treatment against the *rejection* of a *transplant kidney*.

Alpha-blocker A type of *blood pressure* tablet – examples include doxazosin and terazosin.

Amphotericin An anti-fungal drug that combats thrush (infection with *Candida albicans*) in the mouth or gullet.

Angiogram A type of X-ray that uses a special dye to show the *blood vessels*. The dye is put into the blood vessels via a tube that is inserted into the groin and passed up to the *kidneys*.

Angiotensin II (A2) antagonist A type of *blood pressure* tablet, also known as an angiotensin-receptor blocker or ARB.

Angiotensin-converting enzyme (ACE) inhibitor A type of *blood pressure* tablet.

Antibiotic drugs A group of drugs used to treat infections caused by *bacteria*.

Antibodies Substances that normally help the body to fight infection. They are made by *white blood cells*. After a *transplant*, antibodies can attack the new *kidney* and cause *rejection*.

Antibody incompatible transplantation Transplantation in the face of antibodies that could damage the new kidney. AIT involves blocking antibody reactions or removing antibodies using a machine.

Antigen A type of *protein* that occurs on the outer surface of all the *cells* in a person's body. Antigens act as a 'friendly face' for the cells. The *immune system* normally recognises the friendly face of the body's own cells, and does not attack or reject them.

Arteries *Blood vessels* that carry blood from the heart to the rest of the body.

ATG Abbreviation for anti-thymocyte globulin, a strong treatment against the *rejection* of a *transplant kidney*.

Atheroma Deposits of *cholesterol* and other fats that cause furring and narrowing of the *arteries* (also called atherosclerosis).

Azathioprine An *immunosuppressant drug* used to prevent the rejection of a *transplant kidney*.

Bacteria A type of germ. Bacteria are microscopically tiny, single-celled organisms capable of independent life. Most are harmless, but some cause disease.

Basiliximab A drug given by injection at the time of a transplant operation, and again a few days later. Basiliximab blocks the signals that tell *white blood cells* there is a foreign object in the body and so reduces the chances that the body will reject a transplanted kidney.

BK virus A virus that occurs commonly in healthy people and does not cause serious illness. However, it can damage a transplanted *kidney*.

Bladder The hollow, muscular *organ* in which *urine* is stored before being passed from the body.

Blood pressure The pressure that the blood exerts against the walls of the *arteries* as it flows through them. Blood pressure measurements consist of two numbers. The first shows the *systolic blood pressure*, the second shows the *diastolic blood pressure*. Normal blood pressure is 130/80 or less for most people.

Blood vessels The tubes that carry blood around the body. The main blood vessels are the *arteries* and *veins*.

BP Abbreviation for *blood pressure*.

Brain death A term indicating that the entire brain has permanently stopped working. A person must be diagnosed as being brain dead before their organs can be removed for a *deceased donor transplant* from a *heartbeating donor*.

Campath Another name for *alemtuzumab*.

Candida albicans A fungus that causes thrush, which can affect the mouth and throat of people who are on *immunosuppressants* following a *transplant*.

Catheter A flexible plastic tube used to enter the interior of the body. A urinary catheter is used to drain *urine* from the *bladder*, often following surgery or prior to an investigation.

Cells The tiny units from which all living things are built up. Most cells have some common features (including a nucleus that is the cell's control centre, and an outer membrane or skin that gives the cell its shape). Cells in different parts of the body look different from each other and perform different functions (for example, skin cells are very different from blood cells).

Cholesterol A *lipid* (fat) that is a major contributor to *atheroma*.

Chronic A word meaning long term and of slow onset, not usually requiring immediate action.

Chronic allograft nephropathy Another term for *chronic rejection* of a *transplant kidney*.

Chronic rejection Transplant damage that develops slowly, and may be treated with control of the blood pressure, and changes in the immunosuppressant drugs. Strategies include minimising the dosages of tacrolimus or ciclosporin, or switching to mycophenolate mofetil or sirolimus.

Ciclosporin An *immunosuppressant drug* used to prevent the *rejection* of a *transplant kidney*.

CJD Abbreviation for *Creutzfeldt-Jakob disease*.

CMV Abbreviation for *cytomegalovirus*.

Co-trimoxazole An antibiotic commonly prescribed after *transplant*, in order to prevent a type of pneumonia.

Creatinine A waste substance produced by the muscles when they are used. The higher the blood creatinine level, the worse the *kidneys* (or *dialysis* or kidney *transplant*) are working.

Creutzfeldt-Jakob disease A rare infection of the brain tissue that causes dementia. CJD could be transferred from a donor to a recipient with a transplanted kidney.

Cross-match The final blood test before a *transplant operation* is performed. It checks whether the patient has any *antibodies* to the *donor kidney*. The operation can proceed only if the cross-match is negative (i.e. no antibodies are found). If it is positive, *antibody incompatible* treatment might be needed.

CT scan Abbreviation for a computed tomography scan. An investigation that uses a computer to build up a picture from a series of low-intensity X-rays.

Cytomegalovirus (CMV) A *virus* that normally causes only a mild 'flu-like illness. In people with a *kidney transplant* (and in other people whose *immune system* is suppressed), CMV can cause a more serious illness, affecting the lungs, liver and blood.

Daclizumab A drug given by injection at the time of a *transplant operation*, and again a few days later. Daclizumab blocks the signals which tell *white blood cells* there is a foreign object in the body and so reduces the chances that the body will reject a transplanted *kidney*.

Deceased donor transplant A *transplant kidney* removed from someone who has died.

DEXA scan An X-ray that measures the density of the bones. It is used to diagnose osteoporosis.

Diabetes mellitus A condition (also known as 'sugar diabetes' or simply as diabetes) in which there is too much sugar in the blood. Whether this type of diabetes is controlled by insulin, tablets or diet, it can cause *kidney failure*. This happens most often to people who have had diabetes for longer than 10 years. Diabetes mellitus can also be a side effect of some of the drugs used to prevent *rejection* after a *transplant*.

Diabetic nephropathy Kidney failure caused by *diabetes mellitus*.

Diastolic blood pressure A *blood pressure* reading taken when the heart is relaxed. It is taken after the *systolic blood pressure*, and is the second figure in a blood pressure
measurement. It should be 80 mmHg or less.

Donor A person who donates (gives) an organ to another person (the *recipient*).

Donor kidney A *kidney* that has been donated.

Doppler scan A type of *ultrasound scan* (sound-wave picture) that provides information about blood flow through the *arteries*.

Echocardiogram (ECHO) A type of *ultrasound scan* (sound-wave picture) that shows how well the heart is working.

eGFR Estimated *glomerular filtration rate*. The term is generally applied to a test which measures how well the kidneys are working. It is normally around 100 mls/min/1.73 m², which approximates to 100% of normal kidney function. It is similar to the *creatinine* clearance test and is used mainly in the pre-dialysis period.

Electrocardiogram (ECG) A test that shows the electrical activity within the heart.

End-stage renal failure (ESRF) An alternative name for *established renal failure*.

End-stage renal disease (ESRD) An alternative name for *established renal failure*.

Epstein-Barr virus (EBV) The virus that causes glandular fever. It can cause *lymphoma* or *PTLD* after a transplant.

ERF Abbreviation for *established renal failure*.

ESA Abbreviation for erythropoiesis-stimulating agent, a substance which is used for the treatment of anaemia. Many people need to take an ESA while they are on dialysis and waiting for a *transplant*, but it is unusual to continue needing it after a successful transplant.

ESRD Abbreviation for *end-stage renal disease*.

ESRF Abbreviation for *end-stage renal failure*.

Established renal failure (ERF) A term for advanced chronic *kidney failure*. People who develop ERF will die within a few weeks unless treated by dialysis or *transplantation*. These treatments control ERF but cannot cure it. Once a patient has developed ERF, they will always have it, even after a *transplant*.

FK506 Another name for *tacrolimus*.

GFR An abbreviation for glomerular filtration rate, also the name of a test which indicates how effectively the *kidneys* get rid of waste by measuring the number of millilitres of blood the kidneys are able to filter in one minute.

Glomerulonephritis Inflammation of the glomeruli, which is one of the causes of *kidney failure*.

Glomerulus One of the tiny filtering units inside the *kidney*.

Glucose A type of sugar. There is normally a small amount of glucose in the blood. This amount is not usually increased in people with *kidney failure* unless they also have d*iabetes mellitus*.

Graft Another name for a transplant kidney.

Haemoglobin (Hb) A substance in *red blood cells* that carries oxygen around the body. Blood levels of haemoglobin are measured to look for anaemia. A low Hb level indicates anaemia.

Hb Abbreviation for *haemoglobin*.

Heartbeating donor A term used to describe a donor whose heart is still beating after *brain death* has occurred. Most, but not all, *deceased donor transplants* come from heartbeating donors.

Hepatitis An infection of the liver, usually caused by a *virus*. Two main types, called hepatitis B and hepatitis C, can be passed on by blood contact. This means that living donors and *kidneys* from deceased donors need to be screened carefully for these viruses. Care is taken to reduce this risk, and regular virus checks are made on all kidney patients.

HIV Human immunodeficiency virus, the virus that causes AIDS. Tests for this virus are carried out before a patient can have a *transplant*. This is because HIV may be present and inactive in the patient's body but can be activated by the *transplant* and *immunosuppressant drugs*, and cause illness.

Hormones Substances that act as chemical messengers in the body. They are produced in parts of the body called endocrine glands. Hormones travel around the body in the blood, and control how other parts of the body work. For example, parathyroid hormone from the parathyroid glands in the neck affects *kidney* function.

HTA Abbreviation for the *Human Tissue Authority*.

Human Tissue Authority Regulatory body which gives authority for use of any organ from a living donor. The HTA's approval must be given before any living donor transplant can take place.

Immune system The body's natural defence system. It includes organs (such as the spleen and appendix), lymph nodes (including the 'glands' in the neck) and specialist *white blood cells* called *lymphocytes*. The immune system protects the body from infections, foreign bodies and cancer. To prevent *rejection* of a *transplant kidney*, it is necessary for patients to take *immunosuppressants*.

Immunosuppressants A group of drugs used to dampen down the *immune system* to prevent *rejection* of a *transplant kidney*. Commonly used examples are *ciclosporin, azathioprine, tacrolimus* and *mycophenolate mofetil*.

Isoniazid An *antibiotic* used in the prevention of *tuberculosis*.

Kidneys The two bean-shaped body organs where *urine* is made. They are located at the back of the body, below the ribs. The two main functions of the kidneys are to remove toxic wastes and to remove excess water from the body. The kidneys also help to control *blood pressure*, help to control the manufacture of *red blood cells*, and help to keep the bones strong and healthy.

Kidney biopsy Removal of a small piece of *kidney* through a hollow needle for examination under a microscope. It is needed to diagnose some causes of *kidney failure*, including nephritis. It is also used to check whether a transplanted kidney is being rejected.

Kidney donor A person who gives a *kidney* for *transplantation*.

Kidney failure A condition in which the *kidneys* are less able than normal to perform their functions of removing toxic wastes, removing excess water, helping to control *blood pressure*, helping to control *red blood cell* manufacture and helping to keep the bones strong and healthy. Kidney failure can be *acute* or *chronic*. Advanced chronic kidney failure is called *established renal failure* or *ERF*.

Kidney transplant An alternative name for a *transplant kidney*, or for the *transplant operation* during which a new *kidney* is given to the recipient.

LFTs Abbreviation for *liver function tests*.

Lipids Another name for fats. People with *kidney failure* tend to have raised lipid levels in the blood.

Liver function tests (LFTs) Blood tests that show how well the liver is working. They often appear at the bottom of the biochemistry blood test results. Some people with *kidney failure* also have liver problems.

Living related transplant (LRT) A *transplant kidney* donated (given) by a living relative of the *recipient*. A well-matched living related transplant is likely to last longer than either a *living unrelated transplant* or a *deceased donor transplant*.

Living unrelated transplant (LURT) A *kidney transplant* from a living person who is biologically unrelated to the *recipient* (such as a husband or wife).

Lymphocytes Specialist *white blood cells* that form part of the *immune system*.

Lymphoma A form of cancer of the immune system. It can be caused by Epstein-Barr virus in transplant patients.

Malnutrition Loss of body weight, usually due to not eating enough (especially foods providing *protein* and energy). Malnutrition is the major nutritional problem of dialysis patients.

Marker A substance that is known to occur in the presence of another substance. Both *creatinine* and *urea* are markers for many less easily measurable substances in the blood. The higher the blood levels of these marker substances, the higher also are the levels of harmful *toxins* in the blood.

Methylprednisolone An intravenous version of *prednisolone*, a drug used to prevent or treat the *rejection* of a *transplant kidney*.

mmol/L Abbreviation for millimoles per litre. A unit used to measure the blood levels of many substances. *Creatinine* is measured in smaller units called micromoles per litre (μmol/L).

Molecule The smallest unit that a substance can be divided into without causing a change in the chemical nature of the substance.

MRI scan Abbreviation for magnetic resonance imaging scan, a scanning technique that uses magnetism, radiowaves and a computer to produce high-quality pictures of the body's interior.

Mycophenolate mofetil A new *immunosuppressant drug* used as an alternative to *azathioprine*.

Nephr- Prefix meaning relating to the *kidneys*.

Nephrectomy An operation to remove a *kidney* from the body. An open nephrectomy involves removing the kidney by traditional surgical means. A laparascopic nephrectomy involves using 'keyhole surgery' to remove the kidney. A bilateral nephrectomy is an operation to remove both kidneys.

Nephrologist Another name for a kidney doctor.

Nephrology The study of the *kidneys*.

Neutropenia A shortage of *white blood cells*.

NICE Abbreviation for National Institute for Health and Clinical Excellence, and the name by which this body is commonly known. NICE looks at whether new treatments are effective and issues guidelines for good practice.

Non-heart beating donor A donor whose heart is not beating after death, for example after having had a heart attack in casualty when resuscitation has failed. A few *deceased donor kidneys* come from this source.

Nuclear medicine scan Another name for a *radio-isotope scan*. Examples include DMSA, DTPA, and MAG-3 scans.

Obstructive nephropathy Blockage to the drainage system of the *kidney*, through which the *urine* passes.

OKT3 Abbreviation for orthoclone K T-cell receptor 3 antibody, a strong treatment for the *rejection* of a *transplant*. Also called muromonomab-CD3.

Organ A part of the body that consists of different types of *tissue*, and that performs a particular function. Examples include the *kidneys*, heart and brain.

Prednisolone A *steroid* drug used to prevent or treat the *rejection* of a *transplant kidney*.

Proteins Chemical components of the body, formed from amino acids. The body needs supplies of protein in the diet to build muscles and to repair itself.

PTLD The commonly-used abbreviation for 'post transplant lymphoproliferative disease'. This is a form of lymphoma which is much more common in people who have had a *transplant* than in people in the population at large.

Pyelonephritis Inflammation of the drainage system of the *kidneys*, one of the causes of *kidney failure*. It can be diagnosed by an *ultrasound scan*, an intravenous pyelogram or a *nuclear medicine scan*.

Radio-isotope scan A method of obtaining pictures of the body's interior, also called a *radio-nuclide scan* or *nuclear medicine scan*. A small amount of a mildly radioactive substance is either swallowed or injected into the bloodstream. The substance gathers in certain parts of the body, which then show up on pictures taken by a special machine.

Radio-nuclide scan Another name for a *radio-isotope scan*.

Recipient In the context of *transplantation*, a person who receives an organ from another person (the donor).

Red blood cells *Cells* in the blood which carry oxygen from the lungs around the body.

Rejection The process by which a patient's *immune system* recognises a *transplant kidney* (or other transplanted organ) as not its 'own', and then tries to destroy it and remove it from the body. Rejection can be *acute* or *chronic*.

Renal Adjective meaning relating to the *kidneys*.

Renal Patient View An Internet resource where patients can see their blood results and other details of their medical records. Not currently available in all renal units.

Renal unit A hospital department that treats disorders of the *kidneys*.

Renovascular disease Atheroma affecting the *blood vessels* that supply the kidneys ('reno' means relating to the *kidney*, and 'vascular' means relating to the blood vessels). Renovascular disease is a common cause of *kidney failure* in older patients.

Residual renal function (RRF) The amount of kidney function that a patient on dialysis has. This varies from patient to patient. It is likely the RRF will reduce over a period of time, and in many patients, it eventually disappears altogether. A creatinine clearance test is used to assess RRF.

Scan One of several techniques for obtaining pictures of the body's interior without using conventional X-rays. Examples include *CT scans, MRI scans, radio-isotope scans* and *ultrasound scans*.

Sirolimus A new *immunosuppressant* drug which is an alternative to *ciclosporin* or *tacrolimus*.

Sphygmomanometer The instrument used to measure *blood pressure*.

Staphylococcus One of a group of *bacteria* responsible for various infections (often called 'staph' infections). A common cause of peritonitis in patients on peritoneal dialysis, and of line infections in haemodialysis patients.

Statins A group of drugs that reduce lipid levels in the blood, especially cholesterol. Examples include atorvastatin and simvastatin.

Steroid A group of naturally occurring or synthetic substances that include the drug *prednisolone.*

Systolic blood pressure A *blood pressure* reading taken when the heart squeezes as it beats. The systolic blood pressure is measured before the *diastolic blood pressure* and is the first figure in a blood pressure measurement.

Tacrolimus An *immunosuppressant drug*, also known as FK506, which is an alternative to *ciclosporin.*

Tissue A collection of similar *cells* that share a similar function, such as skin cells or *kidney cells.*

Tissue type A set of inherited characteristics on the surface of *cells*. Each person's tissue type has six components (three from each parent). Although there are only three main sorts of tissue type characteristic (called A, B and DR), each of these comes in 20 or more different versions. Given the large number of possibilities, it is unusual for there to be an exact tissue type match between a *transplant kidney* and its *recipient*. However, the more characteristics that match, the more likely a *transplant* is to succeed.

Tissue typing A blood test that identifies a person's *tissue type*.

Toxins Poisons. One of the main functions of the *kidneys* is to remove toxins from the blood (a process known as clearance).

Transplant A term used to mean either a *transplant kidney* (or other transplant organ) or a *transplant operation*.

Transplant centre A special department, part of a larger hospital, which carries out transplant operations. Not all hospitals with *renal units* automatically have transplant centres – some patients have to go further afield.

Transplant kidney A *kidney* removed from one person (the donor) and given to another person (the recipient). Transplant kidneys may be either *deceased donor transplants, living related donor transplants* or *living unrelated donor transplants*.

Transplant operation The surgical operation by which a patient is given a donated *organ*. The operation to insert a *transplant kidney* takes about 2–3 hours. The new *kidney* is placed lower in the *abdomen* than the patient's own kidneys, which are usually left in place. *Blood vessels* attached to the transplant kidney are connected to the patient's blood supply, and the new kidney's *ureter* is connected to the patient's *bladder*.

Transplant waiting list A system that seeks to find the 'right' transplant *organ* for the 'right' patient. It is co-ordinated nationally by *UKT*, whose computer compares patients' details (including blood group and *tissue type*) with those of organs that become available from deceased donors. The average waiting time for a *deceased donor transplant kidney* is about 2 years.

Transplantation The replacement of an organ in the body by another person's organ. Many different organs can now be successfully transplanted, including the *kidneys*, liver, bowel, heart, lungs, pancreas, skin and bones.

Tuberculosis A bacterium that can cause long-term infections.

UKT Abbreviation for United Kingdom Transplant, based in Bristol. This is the national co-ordinator for *transplants* in the UK. It also keeps watch over the performance of other UK transplant centres.

Ultrasound scan A method of obtaining pictures of internal organs, such as the *kidneys*, or of an unborn baby, using sound waves. A device that sends out sound waves is held against the body. The sound waves produce echoes, which the scanner detects and builds up into pictures.

Urea A substance made by the liver. It is one of the waste products from food that builds up in the blood when someone has *kidney failure*. Like *creatinine*, urea is a marker for other more harmful substances. The higher the urea level, the worse is the kidney failure.

Ureters The tubes that take *urine* from the *kidneys* to the *bladder*.

Urethra The body's tube that takes *urine* from the *bladder* to the outside of the body.

Urine The liquid produced by the *kidneys*, consisting of the toxic waste products of food and the excess water from the blood.

Varicella The virus that causes chicken pox or shingles. Chicken pox is usually a mild disease of childhood but it can be extremely severe if it affects someone whose *immune system* is not working normally. This includes people taking *immunosuppressants* to prevent *rejection* after a *transplant*.

Vasodilator drugs Tablets that lower the *blood pressure* by making the *blood vessels* wider, so that the blood can flow through them more easily.

Veins *Blood vessels* which carry blood from the body back to the heart.

Virus A type of germ responsible for a range of mild and serious illnesses. Viruses are much smaller than *bacteria* and usually reproduce inside the *cells* of other living organisms.

White blood cells Cells in the blood that normally help to fight infection. They are part of the *immune system*. After a *kidney transplant*, they can be a 'bad thing', as they may attack (reject) the new *kidney*.

Xenotransplantation The transplanting of *tissues* or *organs* from one animal into a human or other type of animal.

Appendix 1
Kidney disease – what do the numbers mean?

Kidney disease is divided into stages, generally equated with your eGFR (estimated glomerular filtration rate). The eGFR is a measure of how efficiently your kidneys are clearing waste products from your body.

Stage 1	eGFR greater than 90	With some sign (on urine test or kidney scan) that the kidneys are not completely normal but still clearing waste from the bloodstream normally.
Stage 2	eGFR 60–90	With some sign of kidney damage on urine test or kidney scan.
Stage 3A	eGFR 45–59	A moderate reduction in kidney function.
Stage 3B	eGFR 30–44	A moderate reduction in kidney function.
Stage 4	eGFR 15–29	A severe reduction in kidney function.
Stage 5	eGFR less than 15	Established kidney failure, when dialysis or a kidney transplant will be needed.

Appendix 2
Useful addresses and websites

Please note that addresses change from time to time.

British Heart Foundation
Website: www.bhf.org.uk

British Kidney Patient Association
Bordon
Hampshire GU35 9JZ
Tel: 01420 472 021
Fax: 01420 4725 831
Website: www.bpka.org.uk
Provides information and advice to people with kidney illnesses throughout the UK. Grants available.

British Organ and Donation Society
Website: www.argonet.co.uk
Provides information on transplantation and donation.

Cancerlink
Macmillan Cancer Relief
89 Albert Embankment
London SE1 7UQ
Tel: 020 7840 7840
Fax: 020 7840 7841
Helpline: 0808 808 0000
Website: www.cancerlink.org
Helps cancer patients, families and carers with practical and emotional support.

Department for Work and Pensions
Helpline: 0800 137 177
Government information service offering advice on benefits for people with disabilities, and their carers.

Department of Health
Richmond House
79 Whitehall
London SW1A 2NS
Tel: 020 7210 4850
Website: www.dh.gov.uk

Depression Alliance
35 Westminster Bridge Road
London SE1 7JB
Tel: 020 7633 9929
Fax: 020 7633 0559
Helpline: 0845 123 2320
Website: www.depressionalliance.org.uk
Offers support and understanding to anyone affected by depression, and relatives who want help. Has a network of self help groups, correspondence schemes and a range of literature. Send s.a.e. for information.

Diabetes UK
10 Parkway
London NW1 7AA
Tel: 020 7424 1000
Fax: 020 7424 1000
Helpline: 0845 120 29 60
Website: www.diabetes.org.uk
Provides advice and information for people with diabetes and their families; has local support groups.

Employment Opportunities for People with Disabilities
123 Minories
London EC3N 1NT
Tel: 020 7481 2727
Fax: 020 7481 9797
Website: www.opportunities.org.uk

Human Tissue Authority
Website: hta.gov.uk
The HTA was set up to regulate the removal, storage, use and disposal of human bodies, organs and tissue from both living and deceased donors.

Kidney Cancer UK
11 Hathaway Road
Tile Hill Village
Coventry CV4 9HW
Tel: 02476 470 584
Fax: 02476 470 584
Website: kcuk.org
Information and support for people with kidney cancer and their carers. Chat room available via the website.

Kidney Patient Information Websites

www.kidneypatientguide.org.uk
Information for patients with kidney failure, and those who care for them.

www.renalinfo.com/uk
Advice and support for those affected by kidney failure.

Kidney Research UK
King's Chambers
Priestgate
Peterborough PE1 1FG
Tel: 0845 070 7601
Helpline: 0845 300 14 99
Email: info@kidneyresearchuk.org
Website: www.kidneyresearchuk.org
Funds research into kidney disease, its causes and treatment. Works to raise awareness of kidney disease.

Medic-Alert Foundation
1 Bridge Wharf
156 Caledonian Road
London N1 9UU
Tel: 020 7833 3034
Fax: 020 2213 5653
e-mail: info@medicalert.co.uk
Offers selection of jewellery with internationally recognised medical symbol: 24 hour emergency phoneline.

National Institute for Health and Clinical Excellence (NICE)
MidCity Place
71 High Holborn
London WC1V 6NA
Tel: 020 7067 5800
Website: www.nice.org.uk
An independent organisation providing national guidance to promote good health. It provides guidelines for the use of new and existing drugs in the NHS.

National Kidney Federation
From June 2008:
The Point
Coach Road
Shireoaks
Worksop
Notts S81 8BW
Helpline: 0845 601 02 09
Email: nkf@kidney.org.uk
Website: www.kidney.org.uk
Aims to promote, throughout the United Kingdom, the welfare of people suffering from kidney disease or renal failure, and those relatives and friends who care for them.

NHS Direct
England and Wales: 0845 4647
Website: www.nhsdirect.nhs.uk
Speak to a nurse for some common-sense advice about your health.

NHS 24
Scotland: 0845 424 24 24
Website: www.nhsdirect.nhs.uk
Speak to a nurse for some common-sense advice about your health.

NHS Organ Donor Information Service
Helpline: 0845 6060 400
Website: www.nhsorgandonor.net
Provides information about donating organs and how patients can benefit from organ donation.

Outsiders Club
Sex and Disability Helpline
Tuppy Owens
BCM Box Lovely
London WC1N 3XX
Tel: 0707 499 3527 (11 am–7 pm)
Website: www.outsiders.org.uk
A national self-help organisation that helps with sexual problems.

Patients Association
PO Box 935
Harrow
Middlesex HA1 3YJ
Tel: 020 8423 9111
Fax: 020 8423 9119
Helpline: 0845 608 44 55
Website: www.patients-association.com
Provides advice on patients' rights.

Relate
Herbert Gray College
Little Church Street
Rugby
Warwickshire CV21 3AP
Tel: 01788 573 241
Fax: 01788 535 007
Information line: 0845 456 1310
Helpline: 0845 130 4010
Website: www.relate.org.uk
Formerly the Marriage Guidance Council. Offers relationship counselling via local branches, and publishes information on health, sexual, self-esteem, depression, bereavement and remarriage issues.

Renal Patient View
Website: www.renalpatientview.org
This site is currently available through selected renal units only, but in time it will enable all patients to view their own results and care pathways on the Internet.

Renal Registry of the United Kingdom
Southmead Hospital
Southmead Road
Bristol BS10 5NB
Tel: 0117 959 5665
Fax: 0117 959 5664
Website: www.renalreg.com
Collects, analyses and presents data about the incidence, clinical management and outcome of renal disease.

Sexual Dysfunction Association
Windmill Place Business Centre
2–4 Windmill Lane
Southall UB2 4NU
Helpline: 0870 774 35 71
Website: www.sda.uk.net
Association providing help and advice on sexual and relationship problems.

UK Transplant Support Service Authority
Communications Directorate
Fox Den Road
Stoke Gifford
Bristol BS34 8RR
Tel: 0117 975 7575
Fax: 0117 975 7577
Website: www.uktransplant.org.uk

United Kingdom Register of Counsellors
P O Box 1050
Rugby
Warwickshire CV21 2HZ
Tel: 0870 443 5232
Fax: 0870 443 5161
Part of British Association of Counselling and Psychotherapy Regulatory body which provides details of registered counsellors who offer safe and accountable practice.

Vitalise
12 City Forum
250 City Road
London EC1V 8AF
Tel: 0845 345 1972
Fax: 0845 345 1978
Website: www.vitalise.org.uk
Formerly known as the Winged Fellowship Trust, this organisation provides holidays and respite care for disabled people and their carers.

Index

nephrectomy (*cont'd*)
  see also laparoscopic
    nephrectomy; open
    nephrectomy
nephritis, living donors 42
nephrologist 2, 157*g*
nephrology 157*g*
nephropathy
  diabetic 153*g*
  obstructive 157*g*
neutropenia 79, 157*g*
NICE *see* National Institute for
  Health and Clinical
  Excellence
non-directed altruistic donation
  62–4
non-heartbeating donors 23–4,
  157*g*
NSAIDs (non-steroidal anti-
  inflammatory drugs) 118–19
nuclear medicine scan 91, 157*g*
nuclear medicine test, living
  donors 44
numbness in hands and feet,
  causes of 79
Nurofen (ibuprofen) 118, 119

obesity 8, 11, 126–7
  living donors 41, 42
obstructive nephropathy 157*g*
oestradiol 131
OKT3 (orthoclone K T-cell
  receptor 3) antibody 93,
  157*g*
older patients 5–6
open nephrectomy 47, *48*
  compared with laparoscopic
    nephrectomy 49
  pain after 50
  recovery time 47

operations *see* kidney removal
  operation for living donors;
  transplant operation
organ 157*g*
Organ Donor Register 35
orthoclone K T-cell receptor 3
  (OKT3) antibody 93, 157*g*
osteopenia 118
osteoporosis 117–18
  as side-effect of prednisolone
    80
over-the-counter medications
  119

paired donor transplantation *see*
  exchange transplantation
pancreas 112
pancreas transplants 21, 111
paracetamol 118
patient controlled analgesia (PCA)
  pump 50, 72–3
patient information 10–11, 24,
  34–5
  dialysis/transplant decisions
    reversible 2–3, 10
  keeping notes 104–5
  side effects of
    immunosuppressant drugs
    84–5
  withheld 35
patients
  matching kidney to 12–21
  survival 20
PCA (patient controlled analgesia)
  pump 50, 72–3
permission, from donor's family
  35
personality and background, and
  coping with transplant failure
  141–2

Have you found *Kidney Transplants Explained* useful and practical? If so, you may be interested in other books from Class Publishing.

Kidney Failure Explained £17.99
Dr Andy Stein and Janet Wild
The complete reference manual that gives you, your family and friends, the information you really want to know about managing your kidney condition. Written by two experienced medical authors, this practical handbook covers every aspect of living with kidney disease – from diagnosis, drugs and treatment, to diet, relationships and sex.

'The book is, without doubt, the best resource currently available for kidney patients and those who care for them.'
Val Said
Kidney transplant patient

Eating Well with Kidney Failure £14.99
Helena Jackson, Annie Cassidy and Gavin James
If you have kidney failure, you need to adapt and change what you eat. But, as this practical and exciting new book shows, you don't need to go on a crash diet, or to deny yourself the foods you love – you just need to adapt your favourite recipes with kidney-friendly foods.

The authors have provided more than fifty delicious recipes to show you how this works in practice. The recipes have been analysed for their nutritional content and are coded to help you choose the most appropriate dishes for your individual requirements.

Living Well with Kidney Failure £14.99
Juliet Auer
This practical and inspiring book highlights the experiences of a number of very different people, from all walks of life, ages and family situations. These shared personal accounts celebrate the fullness of life that people living with kidney failure can, and do, achieve.

'This cheerful book will be a great help and encouragement to patients and their families trying to become experts on renal failure.'
Dr Christopher Winearls
Clinical Director of the Oxford Kidney Unit

Kidney Dialysis and Transplants: Answers at your fingertips £14.99
Dr Andy Stein and Janet Wild
A practical handbook for anyone with long-term kidney failure or their families. The book contains answers to over 450 real questions actually asked by people with established renal failure, and offers positive, clear and medically accurate advice on every aspect of living with the condition.

'A first class book on kidney dialysis and transplants that is simple and accurate, and can be used to equal advantage by doctors and their patients.'
Dr Thomas Stuttaford
The Times

Type 1 Diabetes: Answers at your fingertips
Type 2 Diabetes: Answers at your fingertips Each £14.99
Dr Charles Fox and Dr Anne Kilvert
The latest edition of our bestselling reference guide on diabetes has now been split into two books covering the two distinct forms of the disease. These books maintain the popular question and answer format to provide practical advice on every aspect of living with the condition.

'I have no hesitation in commending this book.'
Sir Steve Redgrave
Vice President, Diabetes UK

Beating Depression £17.99
Dr Stefan Cembrowicz and Dr Dorcas Kingham
Depression is one of the most common illnesses in the world – affecting up to one in four people at some time in their lives. This book shows sufferers and their families that they are not alone, and offers tried and tested techniques for overcoming depression.

'All you need to know about depression presented in a clear, concise and readable way.'
Ann Dawson
The World Health Organization

PRIORITY ORDER FORM

Cut out or photocopy this form and send it (post free in the UK) to:

Class Publishing
FREEPOST 16705
Macmillan Distribution
Basingstoke RG21 6ZZ

Tel: 01256 302 699
Fax: 01256 812 558

Please send me urgently
(*tick below*)

Post included price per copy (UK only)

☐ **Kidney Transplants Explained** (ISBN: 9781859591932) — £20.99

☐ **Kidney Failure Explained** (ISBN: 9781859591451) — £20.99

☐ **Eating Well with Kidney Failure** (ISBN: 9781859591161) — £17.99

☐ **Living Well with Kidney Failure** (ISBN: 9781859591123) — £17.99

☐ **Kidney Dialysis and Transplants: Answers at your fingertips** — £17.99
(ISBN: 9781859590461)

☐ **Type 1 Diabetes: Answers at your fingertips** (ISBN: 9781859591758) — £17.99

☐ **Type 2 Diabetes: Answers at your fingertips** (ISBN: 9781859591765) — £17.99

☐ **Beating Depression** (ISBN: 9781859591505) — £20.99

TOTAL _____

Easy ways to pay

Cheque: I enclose a cheque payable to Class Publishing for £ _____

Credit card: Please debit my ☐ Mastercard ☐ Visa ☐ Amex

Number _____ Expiry date _____

Name _____

My address for delivery is _____

_____

Town _____ County _____ Postcode _____

Telephone number (*in case of query*) _____

Credit card billing address if different from above _____

_____

Town _____ County _____ Postcode _____

Class Publishing's guarantee: remember that if, for any reason, you are not satisfied with these books, we will refund all your money, without any questions asked. Prices and VAT rates may be altered for reasons beyond our control.